Presenting Mark Russell

Presenting
Mark Russell

☆ ☆ ☆

by Mark Russell

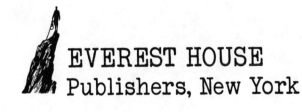

EVEREST HOUSE
Publishers, New York

Library of Congress Cataloging in Publication Data:

    Russell, Mark.
      Presenting Mark Russell.

      I. Title.
    PN6162.R84   1980   818'.5402   80-13197
    ISBN: 0-89696-059-5

The pieces titled "And That Reminds Me..." are based on Mr. Russell's commentaries over the NBC Radio Network and are used with permission of the NBC Radio Network and radio station WRC, Washington, D.C.

for Marie and Marty

Contents

Introduction

"Mark, you're too easy on the bastards."
—NICHOLAS VON HOFFMAN, WASHINGTON POST

"Lay off that Korean bribe stuff, and I'll come back to the Shoreham to see you."
—MEMBER OF CONGRESS

"That vus vunderful—und you are not nahsty."
—HENRY KISSINGER

My act is basically the same as it has been since 1961; only the names, as they say, have been changed to protect the retired and deceased. The trick in doing topical or political humor is to avoid walking well-trodden paths—the forgotten vice president, slow postal service, slow trains, a rich Rockefeller, a cowboy Lyndon Johnson, a talkative Hubert Humphrey, Jimmy's peanuts, Reagan's age, poor Cleveland, flaky California, wintry Buffalo, and so on.

How did Buffalo get its start? They cloned Cleveland. I got my start in Buffalo; my start in life, that is, and to have been born there in the heart of the Great Depression can be perceived as some kind of double-whammy setting you up for anything in life that may come along later. The opposite of such a place and time of birth would be, I suppose, Palm Beach in the twenties.

I have tried to gild the lily a bit regarding the circumstances of my entry into the world by saying, "My parents merely happened to have been in Buffalo at the time—attending the Depression."

Thirty-five years after parochial grammar school, I can remember only five of the seven deadly sins, but that is more than most of my friends who also were taught by the nuns can recall. Usually, at a party, after a few drinks, they can come up with only about three of them—"Let's see, there's lust, greed, anger, (pause), Sleepy, Sneezy, and Doc."

By the time we teens of the forties reached high school, we started to grapple with those sins first hand. Sex education at that time, in an all-male high school run by the Jesuits, consisted of one class I recall, when the teacher, illustrating on the blackboard said, "Now boys, this is the sword and this is the sheath."

My brief college career and my distinguished military service will be dealt with later on, along with an examination of, as my father's favorite magazine *Reader's Digest* puts it: "Life in these United States." One final note of modesty: This book is all you'll ever need to know about me. The story of a lad who went from Buffalo out into The Great Beyond—the Senate, the House, the White House, and network television, but, at the same time, never got out of the Shoreham Hotel in Washington, D.C.

Not that I didn't try. There was the time I went to Spokane, Washington. And here's how *Variety* covered my opening:

> "Mark Russell, whose half-sick humor was something new for Spokane, opened at the Stock Yards Inn last night, and his material was a match for the blue wallpaper and blue table lamps.

> He keeps abreast of the times as he shafts politics, religion, and international affairs. Being a Catholic, he feels free to tell about the waiter who goofed and served a priest Manischewitz wine in a Mason jar."

And so back to the Shoreham. But soon fortune smiled again and I was booked on the old Jack Paar show, but unlike Spokane I never got on. Here's how that event was covered:

> "Bob Hope and one or two other veterans can get away with pot shots at the political greats on TV, but newcomers have to struggle for years to attain that vital public acceptance.

Latest to find out: Pianist-humorist Mark Russell. The producer of the 'Jack Paar Show' called Russell to New York, listened to him, paid him his fee, and sent him back to us."

However, television has since been kinder to me. Realizing that I eventually had to find an honest line of work, I have written this book. Who knows? I might get to like it. It was nice not having even one heckler in my den trying to ruin my act.

Presenting Mark Russell

1. Welcome Aboard

> We hope you understand the reason we must overbook
> our flights. If we don't overbook, the hotels can't over-
> book. —AIRLINE RESERVATION CLERK

Having had a long love affair with aviation, I would still rather not
dwell on the fact that there are suitcases down there in the luggage
compartment with Amelia Earhart's name on them. I honestly
enjoy air travel, and after logging many thousands of miles, I still
have a sense of wonder about defying gravity and cheating death
while soaring, a man-bird, through the clouds.

I am at home in most airports. Washington's Dulles is the most
convenient and attractive, while Atlanta's is the absolute worst in
terms of ugliness and inconvenience. The general atmosphere of
the place can turn the most sunny disposition into a wretched
crank. The design of the Atlanta terminal, with its ever-lengthen-
ing extremities, must have been created by someone who wanted
to teach people a lesson for ever wanting to fly in the first place.
"I'll show them," said the evil architect, "they'll walk as they were
intended to, until they drop."

Atlanta, a world center of commerce, deserves better, but perhaps by torturing so many transients this obstacle-course air terminal stands defiant as Scarlett O'Hara's final revenge.

Why don't the Atlanta transportation authorities come out and
admit that their airport is the perfect location for a movie called
The Doomed Island of the Lost? How about some truth in advertising? Let them put a sign up in the terminal that says, "Welcome
to the Atlanta Airport—Where We Take Pride in Difficulty."
Imagine one of those "you are here" maps of the terminal posted
on the wall; in Atlanta it would say, "You are either here—or
here."

If General Sherman had flown into Atlanta, the Confederacy would have been saved.

Every once in a while on the late, late show, in movies made back in the forties, you can catch a glimpse of America's first busy terminal, at least by forties' standards, LaGuardia Field. Known today, of course, simply as LaGuardia, New York's LaGuardia Field consisted of a modest terminal smaller than the average bus depot of today, decorated in the art-deco style of the time. In the movies you could see William Powell running to greet Myrna Loy as she alighted from a twin-engine antique with aproned wheels, as a stewardess wearing a necktie, severe padded shoulders, and a Joan Crawford harido waved goodbye. Anyone going in or out of LaGuardia was always a millionaire; in those movies, the taxi (readily available, driven by a smiling cabbie wearing a wicker hat, unprotected by a bullet-proof divider) would always deliver Myrna and William, to a penthouse apartment inhabited by servants and white telephones.

That same terminal is still standing, although today it is hidden, off in an obscure corner of the sprawling present-day LaGuardia. The "LaGuardia Field" sign over the doors has been painted over, but the building is still being used as a commuter terminal for passengers of nine-seater aircraft headed for places like Oswego and Elmira. Indeed, it would overload the imagination to picture Myrna Loy or William Powell heading for Oswego.

Named after a mayor of New York who looked like the Costello of Abbott and Costello (and who once read the funny papers over the radio during a newspaper strike), LaGuardia Airport, in the minds of millions of air travelers, is synonymous with the Eastern Airlines shuttle between New York and Washington. Say what you will about the Eastern shuttle, *somebody* has to run an hourly service between these two citadels of fancy finagling, and even though some have likened the trip to a wagon train through Death Valley, at least Eastern took up the challenge. Some of the critics have been mean. Arriving on stage at the Kennedy Center in Washington on one occasion, violinist Itzhak Perlman stood in front of the National Symphony Orchestra dressed in jeans and a yellow sport shirt. The audience, immediately understanding his excuse for not being properly. dressed, roared its approval when Perlman yelled out but two words—"Eastern shuttle!"

The shuttle is convenient, and the approximately one-hour's travel time scarcely allows for movies and champagne, especially since the flight attendants have to collect the fares on board. But there is something about the atmosphere in the shuttle terminal at LaGuardia and aboard the plane itself that turns otherwise nice-looking, pleasant people into haggard refugees. There must be some kind of aging agent in the air or a wizening compound in the water supply, because nobody taking the shuttle looks in the best of health. Or perhaps it has something to do with the evil doings in New York and Washington that most of them are engaged in, and nothing to do with the shuttle at all. On the other hand, people taking the train along the same route appear to be much more robust. I wish I could do something about it—maybe I'll open up a fresh-air camp for the over-shuttled.

There are separate nations within our country. One is called ORD. ORD is, for some reason that escapes me, the airlines' baggage ticket code name for Chicago's O'Hare Airport. Los Angeles is LAX, and Winnipeg is YUG (YUG?), but most baggage codes make more sense. Reno is RNO, Buffalo is BUF, Amarillo is AMA, and Bismarck is BIS. But why would North Platte be LBF? Or Terre Haute be HUF?

There should be more uses for baggage claim checks—kids could trade them like baseball cards. Certainly, a rare BIS would be worth more than a plain old ORD. Perhaps a card game with the claim checks: "I'll see your GEG (Spokane) and raise you one TWF (Twin Falls). As the old saying goes: A MSP (Minneapolis/St. Paul) in the hand is worth two in the YUL (Montreal)." This calls for a baggage check limerick:

> A marriage was failing in HUF—
> The wife said she'd had quite enough.
> So she packed off to RNO and in the Casino
> She met a nice fellow from BUF.

ORD is a land unto itself. As the world's busiest airport, it has more human beings gathered within its confines at any given time than many a town does. ORD should have a mayor and city council because it already has a police department, fire department, church, hotels, restaurants, bars, and even a zoo, which best describes the hordes of transients jamming the terminal itself.

There are a few interesting diversions available to the weary traveler passing through the land of ORD. One of them is to go upstairs to the mezzanine balcony that overlooks the American ticket counters below. This is the one place in the entire complex where one can shut out the noise, because the glassed-in balcony is completely sound-proof. You get a feeling of detachment from the crowd as you peer down onto the masses madly rushing about, in complete silence, in one of the most turbulent spots in the world. There is no reason for the public to go up there; hence the quiet. Other than a couple of offices and a private club run by American, it is a center of solace in a storm of confusion; it also is where the little used, therefore clean, rest rooms are. That there is this vantage place over a troubled world confirms my theory that God is alive and is standing on the balcony in O'Hare Airport.

The cafeterias at ORD are impossible; to clean up after one crowd in time for the next is always an unfinished task. Over in the TWA section they have named the cafeteria the Tartan Tray. Some imaginative public relations person, in an attempt to add a bit of Scottish romanticism to the airport of the city of broad shoulders, as Carl Sandberg called Chicago, came up with that name. Do the busboys wear kilts? Do the bagpipers parade through the cafeteria every hour on the hour? Can you heap your plate with barley, crabs, and sole fresh from the waters of Aberdeen and Dundee? Not by your Firth of Clyde you can't! The total evidence of Scotland lies in the faded design on the plastic cafeteria trays—plaid.

Adjacent to the boiler rooms in the sub-basement of the terminal is the airport's interdenominational chapel. Take the elevator as far down as you can go and you are in subterrestrial ORD. Even a nonbeliever would do well to go down there, if only for a little peace and quiet. But since it is a chapel, unlike the balcony, one can have there a more conventional contact with the spiritual. The chapel is a makeshift affair with about 20 folding chairs and a portable altar, and when it serves as a Catholic chapel it is affectionately known as Saint O'Hare's. I suppose that is because church scholars have yet to confirm the existence of a Saint ORD. The imagination takes over when you are part of the tiny congregation, sitting beneath the crackling steam pipes below decks, receiving the blessings of the chaplain before taking off: "As you go off into the wild blue yonder to lick those Japs once and for all—thumbs up, give 'em hell, and Godspeed."

An eerie wind blows constantly over two rural mountaintop airports which, although hundreds of miles apart, are identical. They are the tiny airports serving Greenbriar, West Virginia, and Vail, Colorado. There is a newer one at Vail (Gerald R. Ford Airport), but I'm talking about the older one perched atop the Rockies. It bears a direct resemblance to the precariously perched runway and log-cabin terminal in the mountains of West Virginia.

These places are worlds away from O'Hare or LaGuardia. Amid complete isolation, one man makes the coffee, processes your ticket, checks your luggage, carries it out to the plane, pulls out the wheel chocks before take-off; and after the plane leaves, I assume, he returns to his chair on the front porch of the terminal to whittle on a piece of wood. In going in and out of fields such as these, the modern-day traveler comes about as close as he can to the barnstorming days of aviation's infancy.

The majority of the airports in the United States fall between the two extremes of O'Hare and Vail. They are the medium-sized ones serving such places as Harrisburg, Raleigh, Rochester, Fort Wayne, Roanoke, Jacksonville, Wichita, and dozens of similar ports of call. Each has taken on a singular drabness of benefit to no one, save the plastics industry, the makers of vending machines, fluorescent tube lighting, and the squeeze mustard container. To be grounded by weather in one of these havens of monotony-by-design is to choose between watching one of those six-inch armrest TV sets, having a coin-operated shoe shine in the lavatory, looking at the proud display of the town's leading industry, or having a spiked rotated hot dog right out of the microwave while waiting for the free bus ride ("surface transportation") to the nearest open airport 165 miles away.

These are the whistle stops of the late twentieth century. Travelers of sixty years ago couldn't dry their hands with automatic hot air; they couldn't get a comb or a nail clipper out of a machine; they never filled out a lost baggage form; a foil-wrapped ham 'n' egger was unknown to them. They never heard the language of flight: "standby," "turbulence," "sickness container," "stacked over Newark," "holding pattern," "return to your seat," and "don't tell any jokes—place all metal objects, coins, etc., into the container before passing under the metal detector." An oxygen mask never automatically dropped down from overhead to be placed directly over the noses and mouths of our poor grandparents as they chugged along aboard the Twentieth Century Limited into Grand Central Station. All the poor things had were dining cars with starched linen, heavy silver service, without benefit of any macadamia nuts.

A few airports, displaying a certain pride, will feature something of distinction that sets them apart from others. There are some that, even though situated deep in the nation's interior, call themselves "international" airports. They may of course qualify for such a global classification because of a weekly mail run coming up from Juarez, but whenever I see signs such as "Welcome to the Enid, Oklahoma, International Airport," I always suspect that they achieved the status by serving English muffins in the coffee shop.

Tampa, Florida, has an airport where easy traveling is something they care about; a convenient little train ride to your plane is a feature that puts the aforementioned Atlanta to shame. My award for the friendliest ticket clerk goes to an unknown lady at the Eastern counter at Boston's Logan Airport. During a three-minute conversation several years ago, she was quite sparkling with a wit and manner that has drawn me back for a quick chat whenever I'm in Boston, but to no avail. I keep missing her, so I'll just think of her as Eastern's Boston Mystery Lady.

The bar at Buffalo's terminal carries Canadian ale—hard to find in an airport. Houston's rotating restaurant is way above the airport norm, although the new terminal itself is dangerously akin to the unspeakable monstrosity next door in Dallas–Fort Worth. Flight attendants were the first to pass the word about the superior quality of the popcorn at, of all places, Dayton's airport. The airport in New Orleans has an excellent oyster bar, and if they could work out an exchange deal with Buffalo, they'd really have something. Miami's outstanding feature is intrigue; passing through its terminal with its proximity to the hot-blooded Caribbean, you know you are not in Fort Wayne, as every third person appears to be bent on hijacking, smuggling, piracy, and various other pursuits of high-handed skulduggery. It's pure entertainment; every time I'm there, I just know that I'll spot Sidney Greenstreet in a Panama suit passing an envelope to Peter Lorre. *The Spirit of St. Louis* hangs from the ceiling in St. Louis, but contrary to the belief of many passers-by, it's a replica. The real one is in the Smithsonian in Washington. There's a nice picture of the late Rhode Island senator Theodore Francis Green in Providence's Theodore Francis Green Terminal—good thing it is there, otherwise it's back to the armrest TV. Most highly acclaimed shoe shine? Cleveland's Hopkins. People around the country are said to mail their shoes to Cleveland for the five-dollar ultraviolet-ray shine. As the song goes, "My Heart May Be in San Francisco, But My Shoes Are in Cleveland." Most awe-inspiring mural? Grand Rapids, Michigan, whose favorite son, Gerald Ford, has his life grandly depicted for the ages along an entire wall. Get stuck in Grand Rapids and you can look at Jerry, Betty, and the kids in various stages of their lives in a panorama of the adventures of the 38th president of the United States.

For the past few years, airports have been serving another purpose besides being points of departure and arrival for those traveling by air. They also have been designated as testing grounds for stretching the First Amendment to the breaking point. Since the mid-seventies, airports have been infested with hordes of pitchmen and pitchwomen, hawking their messages, sermons, pamphlets, and books, attempting to ambush the traveler before he reaches his plane and convert him to Buddhism, Hinduism, Hare Krishna-ism or nuclear power-ism. Frequent travelers know that the only one who can negotiate the open-field running required to successfully dodge all the religious pests in the terminal is O.J. Simpson. (You thought he was renting a Hertz car, didn't you?) They should sell airport insurance which pays for your flight when you miss your plane because some religious zealot won't let go of your hand. If you are late for your plane and at the same time are able to smile sweetly and patiently listen to the pitches of all the Krishnas and Moonies lurking about, you don't need religion in the first place. I'm all for freedom of speech and religion, but whenever I am accosted by one of these beaming cherubs who sticks out his hand

and says, "Hi, there, what's your name?" I find it difficult to refrain from answering, "Diocletian." It used to be that missionaries were sent to places like Africa or India, but now they are sent to work among the natives in darkest LaGuardia.

A Damascus in reverse seems to have taken place at the airports, since the Krishnas have all but disappeared, to be replaced by advocates of nuclear power. Could it be that they are the same people? Is it possible that tiring of the saffron robes, the shaved heads, and the rigors of vegetarianism, they saw the light (or the dark?) and swapped their auras of sanctity for the look of the buttoned-down achievers that their parents hoped for? The Hare Krishna chant has evolved into "Go Nuclear." Agree with it or not, there is something ironic about employing the tactics of the mendicants of Calcutta to praise the virtues of nuclear fission. Come to think of it, India has the bomb—I guess it isn't ironic after all.

Let us turn back to that historic moment in 1903 when Orville and Wilbur Wright started it all. Their crazy stunt at Kitty Hawk was delayed somewhat that day because Orville's monkey wrench activated the metal detector and he had to be questioned by the authorities.

I know the feeling that Orville must have had. Airport security is usually very lax around the world—except when I try to board a plane. If they searched everyone as thoroughly as they search me, hijacking would be ended for good. While terrorists are sneaking firearms of every description aboard airplanes all over the world, my Life Savers are activating the buzzer. It seems that a bazooka is easier to sneak aboard a plane than your car keys. I once saw the authorities stop a sweet-looking elderly lady when they found knitting needles in her purse. The police closed in on her as she shouted defiantly, "Come one step closer and I'll knit right at you!"

Back to the Wright Brothers. During that first flight that ushered in the dawn of aviation, Orville proved to be a typical pilot as he cheerfully pointed out all the places of interest along the route of the 120-foot trip. They made three more flights that day, the longest of which was 852 feet, which is about a third of the walking distance at the average airport today. All in all, it was a near-perfect day for Orville and Wilbur—marred only by the fact that their luggage was lost.

The first airplane cost less than a thousand dollars including a cost overrun of $11.14. Little did the Wright Brothers realize that not only did they invent the airplane, but also a new language, which includes these stirring words: "As we make our final approach into the Kitty Hawk area, please make sure your seat belts are securely fastened and your seat backs and tray tables are in a full, upright, and locked position. Please do not leave your seats until we have come to a complete stop at the ramp and the captain has turned off the seat belt sign. We thank you for flying with Wilbur and myself and we hope you have a pleasant stay here in Kitty Hawk or wherever your final destination may be. Thank you and have a nice day."

The question has been raised as to why Orville was alone as he straddled the wing on that first flight. The only conclusion I can come up with is that Wilbur was bumped.

When the DC-10 crashed during take-off from O'Hare Airport in the spring of 1979, it occurred to me that passengers were now entitled to start making announcements of their own. Upon boarding the plane, the passengers should all recite: "For your safety and our safety, please make sure your seat belts and engines are securely fastened. In preparation for take-off, please see that an eleven-thousand-pound object is fastened to the wing by something more substantial than six three-and-a-half-inch bolts."

Tourists visiting Washington were treated to a sight not listed in their guidebooks on the particular day when a long line of people camped outside the headquarters of the Civil Aeronautics Board with cots and sleeping bags. The occasion was a mad scramble of airline representatives in a first-come, first-serve bid on unused air routes made available by airline deregulation. As at a January white sale at Macy's, they elbowed and clawed to have the distinction of being the only carrier offering a nonstop flight from, say, Nashua, New Hampshire, to Laramie, Wyoming. Some lucky airline would be attracting all those millions of people who travel between New York and Chicago but for some reason must first stop in Altoona. Deregulation gave way to interesting discount plans, some of which were rather complicated: "We offer a 50 percent discount to college freshmen with an SAT score of 1100 traveling with no luggage between Miami and the South Pole on alternative Wednesdays in winter between the hours of midnight and six A.M." I am waiting for a flight designed for people who have seen everything in airline luxury. This would feature a 12-course dinner with champagne and dancing on a 747 flight from Dallas to Fort Worth.

There just isn't enough competition among the airlines. Why not have a low-cost flight for those folks who don't mind standing from New York to Los Angeles? Competition only relates to fringe services as advertised in messages such as: "We're the airline featuring two pats of butter" or "Fly us—we have finger bowls." But how about some real competition? Let's have some rock-bottom prices for those travelers not bothered by having to take their turn at the controls or at the box of kitty litter in the back of the plane where the restroom used to be.

Since airlines are always striving to sweeten the advantages of paying the full fare, I have a few suggestions on how they can make it even more comfortable for those who are not in the chicken-feed section. Full-fare passengers are not given enough choices of seat assignments. All that is offered is first class or coach, smoking or nonsmoking, and window seat or aisle. This is not enough. What if you do not feel like talking to the person sitting next to you? In that case, you should be able to choose a seat in the designated noncongenial section next to a grouch like yourself. But if you feel like having a merry chat, you can ask to be seated in the congenial section. In addition to the congenial and noncongenial sections of the aircraft, they should have the extrovert section and the introvert section. If an extremely shy person is forced to sit next to a life-of-the-party type, his shyness is only magnified and his journey is uncomfortable. But if two shy people are seated next to each other, they will be sensitive to each other and therefore will be more relaxed.

The aim should be to make the flight more comfortable. Therefore, both a liberal section and a conservative section should be available on larger planes. These sections, in turn, should be broken down into liberal Democrat and conservative Democrat, liberal Republican and conservative Republican, isolationist, expansionist, and so on. Insecure sections, smug sections, altruistic

AND THAT REMINDS ME . . .

Jimmy Carter's difficulties in office have raised the speculation that perhaps the presidency is obsolete now that each of us governs ourselves. America has become a nation of more than 200 million separate political parties.

Therefore, we don't need a president to give a State of the Union address anymore, because each of us makes one every day. "I've gotta have gas; that's all there is to it." That's a State of the Union address. "Big government, leave me alone" is another. "We got a hurricane here, and Washington better come through with some money" is yet another. In Texas there actually have been hints coming from the people, including the governor, about seceding from the union, and they sound at least half-serious. "We've got the oil," they're saying, "and the rest of you can all go freeze in the dark."

So we might as well draw up a new Constitution which says: "Me, the people, in order to form a more perfect person, establish justice and a gas tank in my backyard, secure a tax cut for me, but not for the guy across the street, and have my own store that has nonadditive food at 1949 prices, do so ordain and establish this Constitution of the United States of Me."

Our founding fathers could never have imagined the complexities of life in America several centuries later. They were concerned with the basics, such as living and dying. Today, we worry about technology, nuclear proliferation, and dull and dingy hair. If Benedict Arnold were around today, he'd be getting $5,000 a night on the lecture circuit. And he'd be looking forward to the film of his best-selling book. Today our national anthem would be written by Paul Anka as he watched the rocket's red glare and the bombs bursting in air from the deck of the Love Boat. As we secure domestic tranquility by rotating our marijuana crop, let us remember the words of a late twentieth-century mellow Patrick Henry: "I know not what space others may occupy, but as for me, give me liberty or give me my RC."

sections, and selfish sections are also possibilities, but of course this can't all be established overnight. Still, it would be nice to be able to ask for a nonsmoking slovenly window seat in coach.

No salute to flight can conclude without praise for the legendary carrier, Piedmont Airlines. This friendly company has never lost the hospitable spirit of the southern towns it serves, most of them located along the eastern seaboard. The salty tales surrounding Piedmont are mostly of doubtful authenticity; one reported that the airline purchased a Concorde supersonic plane, enabling it to provide more efficient service to Hong Kong, with intermediate stops in Raleigh, Durham, Fayetteville, and Tuscaloosa. In these times of heightened airport security, Piedmont is to be congratulated for the meticulous manner in which all passengers are frisked—the minute they get off the plane. Piedmont passengers are not offered the usual movies, but rather are treated to a more original form of entertainment. After take-off, the copilot wanders through the cabin showing wallet snapshots of his kids, his dog, and his summer cabin on the lake. All in color, and you can view the whole set for only a dollar.

I am indebted to Piedmont for such romantic legends, some of which I, myself, have fostered. I was moved to write a ballad to my favorite airline with a subsalute to her big sister, Delta. The temptation to write such a song came about some years ago when the Top 40 included a tune called "Delta Dawn." Here's my version:

> I prepared to meet my folks down in Atlanta,
> Had that Delta airline ticket by my bed.
> I woke so anxiously, went to the airport speedily,
> But the clerk just smiled, and this is what she said:
>
> CHORUS
>
> Delta's gone, she took off just after dawn,
> Could we arrange another flight instead?
> You can leave without delay, on Piedmont right away,
> So if you've got the courage, go ahead.
>
> I then checked up on all my life insurance,
> And I bought that Piedmont ticket bravely.

For there's only one thing worse, that's Allegheny,
What's good enough for Lindbergh, is good enough
   for me.

REPEAT CHORUS

I sat down and tied the rope that was my seatbelt,
And the stewardess said, "Sir, don't be afraid."
She showed movies, they were colored slides of
   Richmond,
And served two cans of ice cold Gatorade.

REPEAT CHORUS

As we started our approach into Atlanta,
I thought those Piedmont rumors were not true.
But out the window was a sign that bore the greeting,
"Wheeling, West Virginia, welcomes you."

2. Remember When "Energy" Was What You Got in Wheaties?

In the beginning, show business was not in my blood, nor was music, printers ink, or the "theatah." Gasoline was in my blood, if you can believe it. My father worked in a Mobil gas station in Buffalo when I was born. He later advanced to a white-collar job with Mobil, which was then known as the Socony-Vacuum Oil Company. Its trademark of a flying red horse symbolized my earliest childhood. I must have been ten or eleven before I found out that not *all* horses were red with wings. Buffalo is not exactly bluegrass country, you understand. In those days we simply knew nothing of the world, beyond Lake Erie. Come to think of it, I was eighteen before I discovered that Protestants and Jews also played basketball.

For our little family there in the Buffalo wilderness, the flying red horse put food on the table. What was good for Mobil was good for the country. There were no Energy Czars, OPEC, Ayatollah Khomeini, and owning a fin-tailed gas guzzler represented status not stupidity. My father wore the company uniform proudly, and when I grew older, the family nozzle was handed down to me. We were a Mobil family. Had Mobil been the U.S. Army, I would have become Douglas MacArthur.

My brother Dan and I worked for my father in his gas station, and that was the beginning of our present energy crisis. We were both inept. My shoes and socks were constantly drenched with gasoline, since I was totally incapable of filling anyone's tank without running at least thirty cents' worth onto the ground. In those days, thirty cents' worth could drench your shoes and socks. Were it possible to contain all of the gas that I have run over onto my shoes, we could tell the Arabs to go jump into the Persian Gulf.

Just imagine: Geologists searched for a probable place in the earth to drill. Through trial and error they hit one dry hole after another, and then—discovery! The precious crude was pumped out of the ground, and, surging through pipelines, it arrived at the refinery to be processed into gasoline. This gasoline was then shipped to the local distribution point, put into a tank truck, and transported to my father's gas station. Pumped from the truck into underground tanks, the gas awaits its chance to serve—to be pumped once more into an automobile, to achieve finally its noble purpose. A car drives up, and I, the liaison between the public and one of the world's largest global corporations, take the nozzle into my hand, squeeze the trigger—and pour it all over the pavement.

Dan had his own problems. His specialty was to wipe a customer's windshield with the same rag he used to check the oil. People would drive in with perfectly clear windshields and drive out again squinting through a streaky Rorschach test on the glass.

One time, a lady drove in with a very loud noise under the hood of her car. Something was clicking in unison with the rhythm of the engine. As I raised the hood with faked authority, the cadence of the click, click, click grew louder. I called Dan over to the car and said, "Listen to this." He bent over the engine, applied an imaginery stethoscope, and, accompanied by the clicking, started to sing, "Chicks and ducks and geese better scurry, when I take you out in my surrey, When I take you out in my surrey with the fringe on top."

Halfway through the second chorus, the lady headed off toward the Texaco station across the street, with the hood still up.

Our musicianship was further displayed at the station whenever anyone came in with a car having a whistling gas tank. The whistling gas tank was designed to prevent spilling the gas over the top. When you started to fill the tank, it would make a shrill sound that resembled that of a whistling tea kettle. When it stopped whistling, that meant that the tank was nearly full and that you had better ease up on the trigger. If the tank was empty and the owner wanted a fill-up, you could, by alternating the speed of the flow, change the pitch of the whistle and play an entire song. (I should mention that the automatic cut-off nozzle had not yet been invented—nor had self-service pumps, for that matter.) (People who use them seem to be so self-serving.)

Anyway, as I recall (Henry Ford II says this a lot), as I recall, only two makes had the whistling tank—the '49 Chevrolet and a few Packards. The odds were slim that you would have either one of these cars very often for a fill-up.

Dan and I had great fun playing Chevvies and Packards. With two dollars' worth, you might be able to squeeze in "Yankee Doodle." But with a fill-up, which in those days was about $3.50, we played "My Old Kentucky Home" and "Your Cheating Heart." Dan, the better musician, tackled things like "Sophisticated Lady" and "Laura."

One problem was that you had to play the dreamier ballads much faster than they ordinarily would be played, and although it didn't often matter, they were much harder to dance to. Long, sustained notes were impractical, and one time, in a foolhardy act, I spilled over the tank of a Chevvie trying to play "Indian Love Call" on a dollar's worth.

Our greatest musical triumph at the gas station occurred when, against all odds, *two* Packards with extra large gas tanks pulled up for a *fill-up* at exactly the same time. Dan and I tried to remain calm as, nozzles in hand, we prepared for this once-in-a-lifetime opportunity for virtuosity. We had often discussed what we would perform if ever given this rarest of chances. Two Packards in unison needing fill-ups: the Brahms Double Concerto in A minor.

Although it's been nearly thirty years, I'll never forget the harmonies, the counterpoint, the subtle nuances, all deftly played, considering the circumstances. Had this been a performance at Carnegie Hall, we couldn't have felt more artistically fulfilled. And yet, as we silently hung up the hoses, there was no applause, for you rarely get it in a gas station. But no matter. We knew how good we were that day.

The two guys in the Packards probably never forgot that day either. Not because they hadn't the slightest idea of what was going on, but because when they started to pay, my brother and I said, "It's on us."

Ah, but that was long ago. Gas and oil are serious subjects, now that all the Packards, De Sotos, and fin-tailed Caddies have been melted down into Pintos, Gremlins, Chipmunks, and whatever.

Years ago, I began to suspect that maybe the oil companies were deceiving us when they first started putting signs out on the highways that said "Clean Restrooms." While they are drilling for crude, they should also search for soap!

We must keep our hopes up and believe the oil companies will act responsibly with their new-found profits. I believe they have our best interests in mind. I believe they'll plow their profits back into exploration. I believe this will happen on the day Mobil strikes oil in the sports department of Montgomery Ward.

I'm all for free enterprise and diversification. I didn't mind it when an oil company wanted to buy Ringling Brothers' Circus, but if it had, I guarantee that within six months this country would have been suffering from a shortage of clowns—except in Washington, of course. Is our energy problem the administration's fault? Is it Congress's fault? Is it the oil companies' fault? The answer—yes. In other words, I don't think you can separate them. It's like trying to break up the Three Stooges. And now we're told that we're going to have to lower our standard of living. How low? Well, you know the Waltons? They'll be the rich ones. I also believe those who tell us there are seven hundred billion barrels of oil shale deposits locked inside the Rocky Mountains. The big question is: Will we continue kow-towing to the OPEC Countries or will we settle for a flat Colorado?

We're running out of gas because of the Arabs, and because I spilled so much of it. Now the stuff is fast becoming a status product, and to waste a drop can be like dropping a bottle of Chivas Regal Scotch on your way out of a liquor store.

We can expect that magazine ads for energy products will use snob appeal as do the slick layouts for French perfume and gems from Tiffany's:

A butler runs over to the mansion next door and says to the butler there, "Pardon me, old boy, but could I trouble you for a cup of Quaker State?"

The groom slips a diamond on the bride's finger and the caption says, "A diamond is nice, but a cubic foot of natural gas is forever."

Or, "Don't sit home alone again tonight. Put a dab of Sunoco Unleaded behind each ear and say goodbye to Saturday night blues." Or, "Now that you've arrived at the top of the corporate ladder, treat yourself to a quart of Château Arabia '79—an amusing little oil."

Last year, during a time when we were anticipating yet another OPEC price hike, Herblock, the editorial cartoonist, drew a spokesman for the Carter administration speaking to an average citizen. The spokesman is saying, "When they boost oil prices again, we'll swing into action with this." And he is holding up a letter from Jimmy Carter that reads:

> Dear Fellow Americans:
>
> As we said a couple of years ago, we really think it might help if you'd turn down your thermostats and do less driving.
>
> Thank you and good night.

So much for the moral equivalent of war, which is how President Carter described the energy situation in 1976, a year and a half before a semblance of his energy bill was passed.

It took so long to pass it because we couldn't relate to the war that the energy situation was the moral equivalent of. We just didn't feel that old warlike sense of emergency that we felt with Vietnam in the sixties or World War II in the forties. It seemed that certain events would have to take place in order to create the necessary energy-war situation. In other words, unless Jane Fonda joined a car pool, Dr. Spock burned his Exxon credit card and counseled others to do so, and the Berrigan brothers, Angela Davis, Abby Hoffman, and Eugene McCarthy threw themselves down in the streets in front of a gas-guzzling Winnebago, nothing would happen.

Once we Americans are sufficiently aroused, we get the job done, but it always takes a clearly visible enemy before we wake up. It takes a Hitler, unfortunately. In this case, it would take a Tokyo Rose, tauntingly saying, "Hi there, Yank. You're lonely to-night, aren't you? I'll bet right now your best girl back home is running around with some Arab, while you're sitting here with an empty tank."

When the energy bill was finally passed by the Senate, it was voted on along with 24 other pieces of major legislation in a 24-hour marathon. Congress, racing toward adjournment, so that it could go back home and run for reelection, let everything go until the last day, and the energy bill was squeezed in with all the others. When the day was over, one senator was asked to describe the energy bill. He answered, "It has something to do with oil, I know that."

The Department of Energy once made an incredible announce-ment that led me to compare the federal government to Wallace Beery. Wallace Beery was a wonderful old actor; he's no longer with us, but his movies pop up from time to time on the late show, and I just love him.

What the Department of Energy announced is symbolized by the character Wallace Beery played. This was always a warm-hearted but, at times, mean old codger, and there was usually one scene toward the end of the picture where Beery would make a rash promise to his long-suffering wife.

His wife was played by Marie Dressler, and she usually had a name like Old Min. In this scene Wallace Beery would say some-thing like, "Now, now, Min, quit your hollerin'. Ah'm goin' to settle down, you'll see. Why, ah'll quit ma drinkin' and then maybe we can git that little ranch we was talkin' about."

At this, poor old Min would shake her head, knowing full well that the old coot was never gonna change his ways.

And isn't it the same with government? Do you remember during the Vietnam War when Uncle Sam (played by Wallace Beery) said to us, "Someday the war will be over. And when it is, why, we'll take all them billions of dollars we been spending over there, and we'll spend them over here!"

Remember that? And then, a few years later, Ol' Uncle Sam took a slug of red eye and said, "We're gonna build us an Alaska pipeline. And when we do, all that oil is a-gonna come flowin' on down, and they're gonna put it on boats. And then them boats will carry that oil on down here to the lower forty-eight to be redistributed into all our homes and automobiles and nobody, *nobody* can threaten us again!"

Well, they did it, didn't they? Old Uncle Sam kept his promise after all. He built that pipeline, and all that oil, sure enough, came flowing down, just like he said. It's flowing all the time. It's flowing right now, this very minute. And they're putting it on boats, right now. And do you know where the boats are going? JAPAN!

The Department of Energy announced that the oil was going to Japan, and the reason given by its chief (played by Wallace Beery) was that there was a glut of oil on the West Coast.

"Now, Min, quit your hollerin.' We can't get that ranch, you know that. I got the West Coast glut. But things will get better, Min, you'll see. Someday we'll get you that ranch, and we'll have chickens and our own well, and you'll have your very own garden, Min. You'll see."

West Coast glut. Sounds like something you get on a weekend in Tijuana.

Let's imagine another Western movie. This time the main character is bold, upright, the sheriff of the town, his hand steady, always in complete control—Jimmy Carter.

After about ten months in office, President Carter made a tough speech attacking the oil companies, in which he accused the so-called Seven Sisters of "wartime profiteering" and "ripping off " the public. To me, this action was the stuff of a Western classic—a standoff between the sheriff and the villain, Big Oil.

The bad guys in the movie are the Big Oil gang of lawyers, wearing black three-piece suits and carrying attaché cases. The only thing wrong with the shoot-out is that Big Oil owns all the bullets.

"Hold on," says one of the Big Oil guys, "I won't hurt you. I'm here to protect the town from that dirty Arab bandit, Kid Abdul. And if you want protection, I'll need lots of money."

When Kid Abdul threatens the town, the people give Big Oil all the money in the bank. Which is strange, because Kid Abdul *owns* the bank.

So the Big Oil gang and Kid Abdul ride off into the sunset together.

Another version of the plot is found in the following ballad:

BIG OIL

He rode into town with a smile on his face
'Cause a sneer would bring fear to the marketplace.
With his Stetson burnoose and his Brooks Brothers
    suits
And his Gucci cowboy boots he sure looked cute.
Big Oil—Big, Bad Oil.

Nobody knew where Big Oil came from
He just rode into town on a twenty-dollar drum.
Some folks say he came from the Middle East
But he looked like a Texan whose rigs were leased.
Big Oil.

When Big Oil threw his weight around he played with
    fire.
T'warn't long before he raised Sheriff Jimmy's ire.
Folks around town were thinkin' soon
They'd both have a shootout at the stroke of high noon.
Big Oil.

Jimmy rode into town with Jody by his side
And swore he'd give Big Oil a real rough ride.
But how could he know, how could he tell
That Big Oil had seven sisters who were mean as hell.

> There was Esmeralda Exxon, a nasty old dame,
> And Gertie Gulf, from the witch's hall of fame.
> Mabel Mobil and Tessie Texaco,
> If there's a meaner bunch of sisters, man, I don't wanna
>   know.
>
> The clock was approaching the high noon hour.
> How could Jimmy stand up to all of that power?
> But he had a secret weapon strapped to his side;
> If those ladies ever saw it they would run and hide.
>
> Would he use such a weapon on each Seven Sister?
> "Use it!" cried his energy arm twister.
> He pulled it from his holster and nobody could look
> And he shot them all down—with a ration book!
> Big Oil—Big, Bad Oil.

In addition to wartime-profiteering speeches and moral-equivalent-of-war speeches, another way we have attempted to solve our energy woes is the observance of various "days." One of them was "Sun Day," on which talks on solar power were delivered around the country.

The first time they had a Sun Day, I figured a congressional delegation would make a junket to the sun for a first-hand report. I knew the cynic demons really had got to me when I started thinking that everyone in the country working on any energy project actually *needed* the danger of someday running out of oil, coal, and so on. In other words, were it not for the gas lines in 1973-74, we never would have had a Department of Energy. So, all people working at the Department of Energy can thank the Arabs for their jobs.

I guessed that on Sun Day, sun worshipers would gather together and pray to the sun god that the Arabs would keep the price of oil up. Because if it went down, the solar program would go down with it.

How about a Coal Day? On this day, coal miners could gather and offer prayers to the coal god for the oil price to remain high. Because if the cost of fuel oil goes below that of coal, the miners will be home all day watching soap operas.

Perhaps we should have a national Nuclear Day, with nuclear power plant technicians praying to the uranium god for OPEC to stand pat. Because without that need for alternate sources of power, there'll be cobwebs on the breeders. Or a National Energy Day, during which employees of the Department of Energy could pray to the King of Saudi Arabia to continue to frighten us. Why? Because fear means jobs—*their* jobs.

For several years now, the Department of Energy has been having considerable difficulty persuading states to be voluntary burial grounds for excess nuclear waste from the power plants. I can't understand why there is so much resistance. You'd think a state would jump at the chance to be the first one in the union to glow in the dark.

Some people think that the spent nuclear fuel is unsafe, so the Department of Energy is going to launch a campaign to show just how safe the stuff is. Perhaps the latest energy czar could visit each state personally and conduct a demonstration by holding up a Hefty bag filled with plutonium and burying it in front of everybody.

We'll always have those nervous Nellies standing in the way of progress. But thank goodness, Madame Curie went out and discovered radiation, instead of staying home barefoot and pregnant.

It will take some community action to get the program going. It will also take incentive. With a little imagination, a community volunteering to be a dumping ground for nuclear waste could bury it, fill up the hole, and make it into a park, with grass and trees and shrubbery. I think people would come from far and wide to pay admission to see azalias that hum. And pigeons with a dial tone.

Attempting to put this point across, I have been filling the need for a folk singer representing the Big Business side of things. Until now, folk singers always sang about the birds and the trees and the land, while wearing jeans. I walk out on stage wearing the technological folk singer's costume—three-piece pin stripes, the IBM leisure suit. With a respectable piano instead of a guitar, I break new musical ground with these technological folk songs.

This first one can be sung to the tune of "This Land Is Your Land."

> This uranium is your uranium, this power plant is your
>   power plant,
> From California to Seabrook, New Hampshire;
> From the breeder reactor, down in Clinch River,
> This power plant was made for you and me.
>
> Sing of the wonders of our technology,
> And of outmoded powers that it will replace,
> Come gather round the plant and sing our folk songs
> In celebration of atomic waste.
>
> (*and now, a sly little switch to "Polly-Wolly Doodle"*)
>
> Oh, I had an old computer and her name was Clem,
> Sing polly-wolly doodle all the day.
> I got her real cheap down at IBM,
> Sing polly-wolly doodle all the day.
>
> Oh, her digital circuits are a sight to see,
> Sing polly-wolly doodle all the day.
> She's momma's little helper down at ITT,
> Sing polly-wolly doodle all the day.
>
> (*sneaking into "Bury Me Not on the Lone Prairie"*)
>
> Oh, bury me not on the open range
> But beneath the floor of
> The New York Stock Exchange.
>
> Don't wanna hear no cow moans
> From those pastures green
> Wanna hear the Dow Jones
> From Irving R. Levine.

Some time ago, we cut off all aid to Nicaragua because they had failed their human rights SATs. But we continued to aid Iran, even though that country was not squeaky-clean either. But Iran had oil while Nicaragua didn't. That's the way it has to be—unless someone comes up with an automobile that runs on bananas.

When the Shah of Iran had to hightail it out of his country with only the shirt on his back and several billion dollars to his name, we lost a valuable oil spigot. So Carter came up with an emergency, contingency, our-backs-are-to-the-wall plan that included gas rationing. One of the problems with the plan was that each automobile in the country would receive an equal allotment. Everyone in the country would get the same, whether they were a little old lady in Rhode Island who burns up the road once a week to go to church on Sunday, or a rancher in Wyoming with two hundred thousand acres who only uses his car to check on the herd.

The western states complained about the inequity while attempting to increase the speed limit in their states to 65 mph. I guess they felt that was the only way they could legally keep up with the trucks.

Few acts of government have made as much sense as the nationwide 55 mph speed limit resulting from the oil embargo of '73–74. But the theory out West was that if it came out of Washington, there must be something wrong with it. Actually, I think the limit should be lowered to 45 mph. In that case, trucks might slow down to 70 mph.

Everyone agrees that a uniform national speed limit cuts down on confusion. We are one nation and the entire country should keep it at 55. God did not draw up state boundaries. The only reason we need boundaries any more is for football and the Miss America contest.

So let's all do our part to encourage everyone to drive 55. Send one dollar to "Love Our Limit," and we'll put that money to work sending the following message to westerners: You've got a beautiful country out there, so take time to enjoy it. Slow down and hug a prarie dog.

Another difficulty with rationing came up when they started looking for the rationing coupons that had been printed back in '74. Somebody finally found them in a vault at the National Archives along with the WIN buttons and some old Confederate money.

The reaction to the Iranian problem also included turning off all unnecessary outdoor lighting. At the time, I imagined that Congress was certain to modify the plan, making it apply at all times—except at night.

So it goes—one plan after another, as it dawns on us that nobody will make sacrifices on his own. Another big problem will be the inspection of home thermostats. I suggest surprise nocturnal visits by members of the Uniformed Thermostat Task Force. The idea is to catch people by surprise before they can turn their thermostats down. The task force breaks down the door and says, "All right, everybody freeze!" And you must admit it's an easier job than drug enforcement, since the offenders can't flush a thermostat down the toilet.

Turn it up, turn it down,
Whatever the time of year.
We're the Thermostat Task Force
And you'll never know when we'll appear.
You won't know, you won't know,
You won't know when we'll appear.

We're the TTF—surprise!
We're making a random call.
We can tell by the horrified looks in your eye
You were about ready to run to the wall,
But we caught you, we caught you
As you were on the way to the wall.

The TTF is coming your way
To make sure that you comply.
Sixty-five in the winter
And it better read seventy-five in July.
Yes it better, it better
Read seventy-five in July.

The TTF is sorry about
Breaking down your door.
That's the price you have to pay
For the moral equivalent of a war.

So never cheat with your thermostat,
Remember that if you do
My big brother's with the TTF
And Big Brother is watching you!

Keeping our thermostats at 75 degrees in the summer is wonderful news for the several dozen of us who keep them at 68 in winter, as it sort of evens things out. Remember, the magic numbers are 75 and 55. Fifty-five in the building and 75 on the highway. A 75-degree crowded office building—now *that's* the moral equivalent of a war.

Look at all the buildings built for artificially maintained climate control. The windows are sealed shut, and the aluminum and glass exterior attracts enough solar energy to keep the air-conditioning running until Christmas. So what you do is have one problem solve the other. And they're doing it at the Pentagon. They're turning off all the air-conditioners, and those above the rank of captain get a trained specialist to fan them. The fans are your standard government issue cardboard with long wooden poles, painted standard olive drab. Full colonels and above get the best fans of feathered plumes, which you may remember from the afternoon nap scene of *Gone With the Wind*. Incidentally, it is a fact that the Pentagon building is partially heated by an incinerator which recycles the tons of classified material into other paper products. Every once in a while, they find a Russian spy in the building trying to read the toilet paper.

Yes, we in Washington do know what it's like around the rest of the country, because we've had the same gas lines others have had, maybe worse. Perhaps you'd like to hear the gasoline rules we lived with in your nation's capital. To begin with, we had a flag system. Gas stations displayed flags to show the availability of gas for eligible vehicles. A red flag meant no gas. A green flag meant yes—gas. A yellow flag meant only leaded, and a white flag meant the owner had surrendered and was now in intensive care.

We also had odd-even here. As in other parts of the country, if you had an odd-numbered tag you could buy gas on an odd-numbered day. If you had an even-numbered tag you could buy gas on an even-numbered day, except for the 31st of the month when anyone could buy gas, unless he saw a red flag.

Regulations in and around Washington were particularly complicated because of the three jurisdictions of the region—the District of Columbia, the state of Maryland, and three particular counties and five specific cities in the state of Virginia.

Virginia and the District of Columbia each had a five-dollar minimum purchase, but the state of Maryland had a seven-dollar minimum on all cars having six cylinders or more, and a five-dollar minimum on all cars having four cylinders or less. *But* none of this applied to out-of-state cars, ambulances, mopeds, and (they were very particular about this) *professional* funeral vehicles. (What an amateur funeral is, I don't know. And I don't want to find out.)

I guess this meant that a hearse could cut into the gas line any time it wanted, but the rest of the procession could not. Since it follows that a funeral is usually three days after you go, if you die on the first of the month, you had better hope that your friends who need gas have an even-numbered tag. Except, of course, the mourners who show up with out-of-state mopeds.

In the wake of the gas shortages, Washington came up with another new plan: Odd- and even-numbered secretaries of energy. How did we tell them apart? Well, the even Secretary of Energy was the one with the pipe. When James Schlesinger was Secretary of Energy, he was so even that when he took two short puffs on his pipe in rapid succession you knew he was hysterical.

And did you know that there was an energy hotline? They wanted to hear all your responsible questions about energy, like "How come the guys at the gas station won't check my tires any more?" and "Are electric pencil sharpeners unpatriotic?" The Department of Energy had second thoughts about its hotline, however, and couldn't decide whether to give it an unlisted number or transfer the calls to Dial-a-Prayer.

I thought the energy hotline was a great idea. I mean, where else could you pick up the phone and vent your angers and frustrations over a direct line to a powerless switchboard operator? This had the same effect as sending an obscene mailgram collect. Former Secretary Schlesinger, himself, once took a few calls on the hotline. A man called in screaming that every time he drove his car, he felt that he was being gouged by the ripoff prices at the gas pump. Schlesinger puffed on his pipe and replied, "Stay home."

The annual answer to the gas shortage is, of all things, busing.

You have to sympathize with all those teachers who each year must explain to their students why we have gas shortages and busing at the same time. Theorists will tell you that the two issues are unrelated, probably because they believe that school buses run on jelly beans. I modestly submit that no discussion of busing is complete without considering Russell's Laws of School Transportation.

LAW NUMBER ONE: Students are wiser today, only because it takes them so long to travel to school on a bus. They are much older when they get there; therefore, they are wiser.

LAW NUMBER TWO: People's enthusiasm for busing is in direct proportion to the number of children they have at home who are over 22 years of age.

LAW NUMBER THREE: In the city of Cleveland, the people can be inspired to accept busing cheerfully only if their mayor sets an example and moves his office to Detroit.

LAW NUMBER FOUR: Busing would have had a better chance in Cleveland if the ex-mayor Dennis Kucinich had set an even better example and rode the bus with the other kids.

Busing is the law. Congress recently voted to uphold it, which brings us to

LAW NUMBER FIVE: The length of a politician's speech praising the virtues of busing is on a sliding scale with the number of children he has in private school.

You might be interested to know that during the gas shortages, House Speaker Tip O'Neill, Majority Leader Jim Wright, Minority Leader John Rhodes, Senate Majority Leader Robert Byrd, and former presidential candidate Howard Baker all bought gas at a secluded, special VIP gas station near the Capitol for 67 cents a gallon.

Your initial reaction to this might be outrage, but remember the sacred motto of our Republic: "Rank has its privileges." The fact is that 67 cents a gallon is far too high a price. We must realize that a limousine gets less miles per gallon than a Toyota. So doesn't it follow that these congressional leaders should pay less? These are our exalted rulers. Does the Queen of England go to the laundromat? Does the Emperor of Japan carry the trash cans out to the sidewalk? Look at the Pope; do you see the worship and adulation he receives? I ask you, should Howard Baker receive any less? Whatever happened to respect? Whatever happened to honor? Whatever happened to 67 cents a gallon?

Congress and the administration seem to be having trouble agreeing on which version of gasoline rationing is best—allotments of coupons to states according to the number of registered vehicles, or according to the amount of fuel consumed. Well, not to add fuel to the fire, I hereby offer additional rationing guidelines for their consideration.

PLAN A: All motorists living in Wyoming will receive extra coupons if they move to Rhode Island.

PLAN B: Every driver in the nation must write a 200-word composition titled, "Why I need more gas than anybody else." A board of judges will distribute coupons based on originality. Remember, neatness and spelling count.

PLAN C: Families with four cars get no coupons for that fourth vehicle, unless that vehicle is a hearse.

PLAN D: Little old ladies owning 1946 Hudsons only driving them to church on Sunday will receive the minimum number of coupons, unless after church they compete at the local drag strip.

PLAN E: This is used mostly in Washington, D.C., and applies to diplomats from OPEC countries. Under this plan, a form letter is sent from the gas station to the embassy. It says, "Don't call us; we'll call you."

But the House leadership should know that there is only one fool-proof way to guarantee passage of any gas rationing plan—attach it to a Congressional pay raise.

As I said earlier, we Americans can do the job, but not until we are shocked into doing so. We need that visible symbol of the enemy, and I think I've found it. It's the disease of gasoholism. Now you know how riled up we get when it comes to fighting a disease. If you don't, you've never heard of Jerry Lewis.

That car of yours sitting out there is sick, and if the poor wretched thing could talk, here's what it would say:

"At first, I wouldn't admit to it, but now I am willing to face the truth. I am a gasoholic. The energy crisis has made it easier for many of us cars to come out of the garage and admit that we are gasoholics. What causes our condition? We are driven to it. I got hooked on the stuff at an early age. I've quit before, but when I do, I don't seem to have the energy to leave the house. Thank goodness we have finally come around to learning that gasoholism can be cured. How? One day at a time."

3. Show Biz! Movies! Glamour! The Federal Reserve!! and Much, Much More!!!

Kid, I'm gonna make you a star.
—WARREN G. HARDING

Say what you will about old Lyndon Baines Johnson. He may have walked the land as a caricature of wily craftiness, but on the plus side, he left behind two fine men who couldn't have been closer to the old codger had they been his own sons—Jack Valenti and Bill Moyers. They have contributed to our cultural enrichment in a way LBJ never could. Valenti, a former ad-man and Moyers, a former Baptist preacher, both native Texans, first appeared in Washington around twenty years ago as nondescript cogs in the Johnson entourage. But with the influence that came from their White House association, they pulled ahead of the faceless federal pack and emerged as members in high standing of the Washington, D.C. branch of Beautiful People, Inc.

Unlike some veterans of past administrations, Valenti and Moyers were unscathed by their Lyndon Johnson connection, probably because they had the good sense to quit their jobs just before body counts and napalm and Ho Chi Minh made the White House a most unpopular place. Today they are respected and popular figures in the glamorous world of—of all things—show business.

As president of the Motion Picture Association of America, Jack Valenti serves as a link between the movies and Washington. With offices a block away from his old desk at the White House, he is an island of Hollywood glitter in a sea of bureaucratic drab. Flawlessly tailored and barbered, his suave manner graces any hostess's guest list with a charm that is still Texan, but with more jet-age Houston than Johnson City in it.

Valenti gave us the movie rating system, which, although controversial, is a step out of the dark ages of the old Legion of Decency. Considering that Washington meddling in our motion pictures could have resulted in a much more complex rating system than the one we have, I suppose we're lucky and should thank Jack Valenti. When the ratings were first instituted, we feared the worst: rated G, rated PG, rated R, rated X, and—who knew— rated V, those under 17 must be accompanied by Jack Valenti.

Bill Moyers, a bit more subdued but equally debonair, has created and hosted some of the most critically acclaimed TV documentaries, the sort referred to by anyone wishing to make the point that, yes, there are *some* good things on television. So rest easy, Lyndon—you took the Moyers boy out of Texas, and with your help, he made himself into a Lone Star Alistair Cooke, the ultimate sophisticate, who on one day sips champagne with David Rockefeller in a three-star restaurant in Europe and on another, shows his viewers the saintly life of Dorothy Day running a soup kitchen in the Bowery. Valenti and Moyers prove that you can be a part of Washington's contribution to entertainment without being elected.

A perfect example of the Washington-Show Business alliance is the placing of Archie and Edith Bunker's old worn-out living room chairs on permanent display in the Smithsonian Institution. "All in the Family" deserved to be dignified by our most famous museum. Perhaps future space in the Smithsonian could be reserved for other artifacts of television. Tourists may one day line up for a peek at Howard Cosell's toupee, bronzed for all time in a plexiglass case, or perhaps a buffalo chip from "Bonanza" right next to the moon rock. I personally would like to see a bit of permanent memorabilia from the long-time favorite "Sixty Minutes." I'm thinking specifically of two "horsefeathers" and a "poppycock," once spoken to Shana Alexander by James J. Kilpatrick.

As Washington occasionally takes on a Hollywood air, the reverse is bound to happen, and events in movieland will become more characteristic of the capital city than of Tinsel Town. They've already had occasional financial scandals at the big studios, and NBC in Burbank once went into turmoil over a government-style leak to the press. This occurred when someone connected with the "Tonight Show" let the story leak to the press that Johnny Carson wanted out. This was the last thing NBC wanted to happen. Not only Carson's departure, but even hints that he wanted to go, would have a terrible effect on their already poor ratings. Such was the effect of the leak that this breach of security became the Burbank version of the Pentagon Papers.

Everyone working in the NBC buildings in Burbank and New York assumed that they would be placed under house arrest until the leaker was found. Punishment would be severe: six months tied to a chair watching old tapes of "Tonight Show" substitute hosts with nothing but bread and water—which in California means Perrier and Wheat Thins.*

Hardly a person in this country can remember a time when there was no "Tonight Show." When I was a kid, we felt the same way about FDR. But alas, eras eventually fade from the scene. Al-

---

* Critics agree that of all the substitute hosts, the most entertaining, intelligent, and witty one is Kermit the Frog.

though the Carson show is an institution, it is not provided for in the Constitution. Show me where our founding fathers wrote: "We the people of the United States, in order to form a more perfect union, will be subjected nightly to three people on a couch, and one at a desk, accompanied by a trumpeter in funny clothes." Washington-as-Hollywood is a natural evolution with a visibility higher at some times than at others. A Watergate or an ABSCAM is delightful live theatre, and various attempts to reproduce such spectaculars on film or video tape always result in a lesser product. *Mr. Smith Goes to Washington,* made in the thirties with Jimmy Stewart starring as a clean senator who couldn't be bought, probably seemed authentic at the time. People didn't flock to visit Washington as they do now, so that I'd doubt if anyone cared whether the Senate chamber was rarely the turbulent, suspense-filled, brawling arena depicted in the picture.

One of the most hilariously inauthentic scenes I ever saw in a movie about Washington was in *Advise and Consent.* In this early sixties offering, a president dies but his vice president doesn't know it. As vice president, he is presiding over the Senate, which, although provided for in the Constitution, he seldom ever does. In the movie, he has now become the president. This is dramatized by two dozen secret service men marching down the marble corridor in lock step, wearing identical pork pie hats to tell him. The only thing missing was the agents breaking into a song by Gilbert and Sullivan.

Let us examine a few movies about life in the citadel of democracy, some of which were regular movie movies and others especially made for television. In no particular chronological order, they are *Washington Behind Closed Doors, Grandpa Goes to Washington, Eleanor and Franklin, The Seduction of Joe Tynan, Blind Ambition,* and *All the President's Men.*

"Washington Behind Closed Doors" was ABC's five-episode drama about a president who, having gotten himself into a tangled web of mistrust, suspicion, and corruption, faces the possibility of being driven out of office. The president's name was Richard Monckton, and the show was adapted for television from a book by someone named John Ehrlichman. Well, I don't know who this fellow Ehrlichman is, but I'm afraid he let his imagination get the best of him. Were he to ever live in Washington, he would see that such a plot as the one concocted in his book just simply stretches all bounds of reality. Such things couldn't possibly happen in a constitutional democracy, and to portray my city as a haven of cunning and malice is something to which I take personal exception as a patriotic American.

But fiction is fiction, and I suppose there is nothing to stop some money-hungry film maker from doing a miniseries about a president named Jimmy Darter. And since we are fantasizing, ABC could try and get the actor Raymond Burr to play the part of Burt Glance. The point is that anyone who fell for ABC's fictional line of bunk just doesn't know Washington. But some of us do—and we still miss Ike.

At the beginning of the 1978–79 television season, CBS launched what they hoped would be a rollicking romp about life in that wild and crazy place, the United States Senate. The star of the series, called "Grandpa Goes to Washington," was the veteran actor and song and dance man Jack Albertson, playing the part of a man from California who, in his later years, runs for the Senate because he's mad as hell and can't take it anymore. Grandpa gets elected, goes to Washington, and, as they say in the TV listings, "hilarity ensues."

"Grandpa" barely made it through the first 13 weeks of his term in office, and here is my review written after the show premiered:

> "Grandpa Goes to Washington," one of the TV season's new shows, exemplifies what kind of senators we would have if all the voters were comedy writers living in California. The lovable senator portrayed by the lovable actor Jack Albertson wisecracks his way through the show freely dispensing the lovable kind of crowd-pleasing bromides that Hollywood thinks is what elects senators. I guess Jack Albertson got the role because Howard Jarvis can't tap dance.

The first of the "Grandpa" series dealt with sex, graft, blacks, Indians, and a politician's affair with a stripper named Boom-Boom Brasilia. They covered it all in the first show, and supposedly they had 12 more to go. So, the writers had two choices. They could do an episode on each of the aforementioned subjects, or they could show what the United States senator's life is really like 98 percent of the time. Such as: Grandpa goes to the finance committee and helps mark up H.R. 13511. Or Grandpa attends the Joint Economic Subcommittee hearing on priorities and budgeting effects on the proposed ship-building claims settlements and Navy procurements. After which Grandpa will say, "Hey, do you guys know 'Melancholy Baby?' "

A year or so later, a much younger senator was portrayed in movie theatres around the country and seemed to capture our imaginations more successfully than did Grandpa. This time, Senator Joe Tynan, played by the very popular star of "M*A*S*H," Alan Alda, revealed to the public that senators have sex lives. Where Grandpa only talked about it, Joe Tynan is one of those public servants who is a doer and not just a talker. After seeing that movie, I wrote this review:

> *The Seduction of Joe Tynan* is just one more example of what Hollywood's image of Washington is. This film stars Alan Alda, Meryl Streep, and Barbara Harris. Alda plays a United States senator who, you'll recall, had been a wisecracking army doctor who did Groucho Marx impressions in Korea. Harris is the weary Senate wife who, after analysis, takes care of their screwed-up children all by herself because the senator is a driven, power-mad politician whose colleagues in the Senate break a lot of commandments, particularly the ones about drinking and coveting.
>
> Even Alda has an affair with Meryl Streep. Meryl Streep is very beautiful. The only problem I have with Meryl Streep is pronouncing her name. So Barbara Harris finds out about Meryl Streep and calls her the worst name she can think of—she calls her Meryl Streep. Now *there's* a big domestic argument. Barbara starts throwing things at Alan, and he has to use everything he has at his senatorial command to defend him-

self. First he hollers, "Point of order, will the wife yield?" That doesn't work, so he does his Groucho Marx impressions, but Barbara threatens to leave him unless he straightens out. So, according to this Hollywood version, Washington—with its drunkenness, adultery and vice—is a typical average American town after all.

As part of the Bicentennial flavor of the televised historical offerings of the time, ABC announced a docu-drama to be called "Eleanor and Franklin." Since it was on ABC, suspicions naturally arose as to how the network would treat these two figures. Irreverent speculation surfaced as to whether FDR's long-time association with Lucy Mercer would be included (it was), and, if so, would this turn out to be a thirties version of "Three's Company." As it turned out, the series wasn't bad, but I had feared the worst and wondered if ABC would, while plugging "Eleanor and Franklin," pull out all the stops in the PR department:

> ABC, the network that gave you "Charlie's Angels," "Happy Days," and "Laverne and Shirley," proudly presents "Eleanor and Franklin." Tune in and turn on to Hyde Park hijinks with those happy-go-lucky Roosevelts! On the season kick-off, your sides will split when little Elliot brings home a frog and drops it down sister Anna's dress! And you won't want to miss next week when Eleanor puts her foot down after Winston Churchill falls into the punch bowl and sticks his cigar into the mashed potatoes! Starts Monday—right after "Abe and Mary Lincoln Go to Las Vegas."

Television soon returned to a more current time in Washington with "Blind Ambition," the story of one of the capital's swashbuckling sex gods, that heart throb of the cocktail party circuit, John Dean. This was the story of an earnest-looking, power-hungry lawyer who wears glasses and a three-piece suit. And who has a problem—he looks like everyone else in Washington. But, in the movie, John Dean has a secret power: When he goes into a phone booth and removes his glasses, he comes out looking like a handsome actor who can overthrow presidents and romance tall blonde girls.

"Blind Ambition" gave rise at the time to predictions that the Washington lawyer would be the season's newest TV hero. The time seemed right for a pilot script about a restless attorney who burns his Brooks Brothers suit, throws his attaché case into the river, grows a beard, and takes up a new life in the wilds of New Mexico. The working title was "Grizzly Ehrlichman."

G. Gordon Liddy's TV appearances in the spring of 1980 recalled Watergate and provided a refreshing distraction from the daily doses of inflation, Iran, and the presidential campaign. NBC was thrilled about what a smash Liddy and E. Howard Hunt were on the "Today Show." It was the network's finest hour that season, if you don't count the night a duck on "Real People" yodeled "Some Enchanted Evening" through at least three bodily orifices. Liddy told Tom Brokaw on the show that his heroes were Julius Caesar and General Patton, as if we expected Mister Rogers and Truman Capote. Liddy admitted that he was once prepared to murder Hunt. He said it was all in his book. Then Hunt came on the show and was so mad that he forgot to mention his own book. Then Liddy moved across town to "Good Morning, America" and said he had been prepared to murder Jack Anderson. He said that was in his book, too. Then Anderson came on and shook Liddy's hand, which was very painful because Liddy was holding a flame under his hand at the time. ABC was delighted with the show and invited Liddy back sometime to shoot David Hartman. NBC started working on a series for Liddy and Hunt—perhaps as co-hosts on "The Newly Dead Game." Liddy said his image of brutality had been overplayed, that he liked nothing more than to relax with a good book by the fire—all right, *in* the fire. He's really a pipe-and-slippers kind of guy—lead pipe and hobnail slippers. I think the word for Libby is "poetic"—a loaf of bread, a jug of wine, a case of grenades, and a bed of nails.

All the President's Men was one of the better Washington-based movies. Its director, Alan Pakula, seemed to be going in the same direction as the authors, Bob Woodward and Carl Bernstein, who, as the reporters responsible for exposing Watergate itself, could hardly permit themselves to be tainted with Hollywood falseness. Although the *Washington Post* scenes were shot in Hollywood, the desks, chairs, trash cans, and even the trash itself at the *Post* were carted out to the Coast for authenticity. In fact, one of the

real reporters, Phil Casey, expressed worry that future generations
would go to a drive-in movie and see his old love letters up there
on the screen. But the deftest touch of authenticity was in the
casting of the part of the editor, the tough, macho, shrewd Ben
Bradlee. He was brilliantly played by the tough, macho, shrewd
Jason Robards, Jr.

The only trouble with *All the President's Men* was that it dealt
with just a small portion of the Watergate story. Woodward and
Bernstein's book was mainly concerned with tracing the break-in
to the White House. Watergate's subsequent revelations were dramatized only in the previously mentioned television movies. *All
the President's Men* contained nothing of the Sam Ervin hearings,
John Dean, John and Martha Mitchell, hush money or dirty tricks.

It is only now that we know so much more of the story that we
can image the much broader theatrical possibilities of a film about
all of Watergate.

First of all, it would have to be a musical. As the movie begins,
we see a vast football stadium filled to capacity with all the people
in government who are implicated in the Watergate crimes. Richard Nixon, still very much above the battle, comes out in the middle of the field and with a wave of the hand grants executive privilege to the crowd, as the chorus sings a White House memo set to
the melody of "The Teddy Bears' Picnic."

> If you go up to the Hill today, you better go in disguise.
> If you go up to the Hill today, it's a thing that wouldn't
> be wise.
> The President's orders are perfectly clear,
> Your job will be gone when you get back here.
> So hold your tongue cause you've got executive priv-
> ilege.
>
> They're closing in now and getting too close because of
> the Watergate.
> And if you are captured try not to crack even though
> you are burned at the stake.
> Don't talk to reporters, not on your life,
> If you want to see your kids and your wife.
> Some call it a threat, we call it executive priv-ilege.

In another scene, we see the busy workers diligently toiling away at the Committee to Re-Elect the President (CREEP). The members of the CREEP chorus move to center stage for this stirring ballad:

> Working all day on the campaign committee
> It's part of the Washington scene.
> Before you go home at night, clean off your desk
> And throw it in the shredding machine.
> Throw it in the shredding machine.
>
> Rip it up, chop it up, shred it up, and grind it up.
> Papers, candy wrappers, leave none.
> Don't let nobody get it, when in doubt shred it,
> Or you'll read it in Jack Anderson.

As clouds of suspicion descend over the White House, tension tightens in the Oval Office and the presidential staff is summoned to an emergency prayer breakfast. Billy Graham, as the White House chaplain, offers a prayer in solemn tones:

> We thank thee, Father, for thy blessings and for Executive Privilege. We ask you to look down upon the Great Kingdom of the United States and our King Richard who watches over his people with the kindly council that what they don't know won't hurt them. We ask you to bless Sony, whose electric devices are placed upon the telephones of the evil ones. Grant us that our good king may continue in his vow of silence. Father, we implore thee to chastise the misguided Philistines who dwell on the Capitol Hill of Perdition; that they will mend their evil ways and seek no more to learn those truths which are ordained to be locked behind the walls of this Great White Palace forever. And that the guardian of those truths, King Richard, will be able to still the tongues of the erstwhile fink, Prince Dean. We ask that our prayer be answered, lest the truth leak out and the kettle overfloweth and the beans spilleth, because for us, O Father, that would truly be Hell. Amen.

The action switches to downtown Washington, and we see the shadowy figure of former Attorney General John Mitchell sneaking into the office of the famed attorney Edward Bennett Williams. A reporter from the *Washington Post* spots Mitchell and asks him what he's doing there. Mitchell snarls "picking up my Redskins season tickets." The reporter then asks Mitchell what he knows about Watergate and he answers, "None of us had anything to do with it, nor do we know anything about the bugging activities . . . activities . . . activities . . . activities." But the reporter continues to dig and prod, and finally, in one of the movie's most dramatic lines, taken directly from actual newspaper files, John Mitchell says, "I don't know anything about all that crap."

That evening, in their living room at the Watergate apartment, John says to his wife, "Martha, you're not going to tell 'em about the crap, are you?"

MARTHA: I know more about the crap than you think I do, John.

JOHN: That's a lotta crap, Martha, you leave my crap out of this.

MARTHA: I'll talk about any crap I want to, John.

JOHN: Oh, crap.

MARTHA: Don't you 'Oh, crap' me! If it wasn't for me, you'd still be working for those people. They can't fire you if you haven't worked in six months.

JOHN: I know, Martha, but I could go to jail.

MARTHA: Well, do me a favor before you go.

JOHN: What's that?

MARTHA: Have the phone put back in. In fact, you can do it yourself. You always were a good wire man.

We come now to the high point of the film—the president's press conference. Nixon is still stonewalling, but murmurs of impeachment are growing louder. The president has just declared that he is not a crook, and as the Marine Band and the Mormon Tabernacle Choir softly render "America the Beautiful" in the background, he continues:

Oh, I could tell you all I know about this little caper, but that would be the easy way. It's national security that I'm worried about. What's more important, it's my security that I'm worried about. But, I'll tell you this—impeach me and you impeach everything that is good about America. Impeach me and you impeach Abraham Lincoln. Impeach me and you impeach the members of my immediate family—Bob Hope, John Wayne, Billy Graham, and Sammy Davis—in that order, of course. They've been a real comfort to me through all of this, believe me. John Wayne said he would walk into the sunset with me any time. And let me tell you what Sammy Davis said. He said, "Hey, baby, right on, I can dig it, man." Billy Graham gave me some solid spiritual advice—he told me to lie like hell. Impeach me and you impeach station wagons, Lawrence Welk, and the Dallas Cowboys. Impeach me and you wipe out the Boy Scouts, slurpies, Sunday school picnics, and the entire state of Kansas. We did what we had to do for a reason. We learned that Democratic chairman Larry O'Brien was planning to kidnap Mamie Eisenhower. Now, I could not let that happen to my daughter's mother-in-law.

As the music comes up to full, the entire press corps is sobbing uncontrollably, except for David Frost, who is in the back of the room, furtively taking notes.

The sordid drama reaches its climax in the resignation and the swearing in of Gerald Ford. In the final scene, some months later, Nixon looks up from his memoirs and in a reflective, poignant mood, gazes out the window overlooking the rolling waves, tumbling up onto the San Clemente shoreline. Casting a quick glance at the presidential seal on the breast pocket of his pajamas, to the melody of "The Way We Were," he slowly sings:

Mem-ries, of my happy White House days
In my first administration,
Oh, the way we were.

Paris peace talks, Julie's wedding, Chinese trip,
Back home to a grateful nation,
Oh, the way we were.

AND THAT REMINDS ME . . .

At Fort Knox you get much faster service if you are in the eight packages or less express line.

There's a lot of talk these days about the price of gold finally getting up there close to $600 an ounce. Well, that doesn't bother me because I couldn't afford it when it was only a lousy $250. The thing about gold is that it's just as scarce and limited in its supply as, say, oil. But you don't see jewelry stores closing down at noon. And when gold finally reaches $600 or more, just wait, there won't be any more of it around than there was before. And you know why—because there is no gold OPEC. Now, the thing I like best about gold is that we don't need it. Six-hundred-dollar gold fills a tooth just as well as fifty-dollar-gold. And you'll never see odd-and even-numbered charm bracelet lines. Okay, I admit it. Yes, I am sad about gold being so expensive. It's going up almost as fast as beef. Takes a lot of gold to buy beef. And chuck steak is so expensive, they ought to call it "Charles." I like gold, and I love beef. So, I did the only thing I could do. I bought an ounce of chopped chuck, took it to a jeweler, and had it made into a ring.

Happy days with Bebe Rebozo,
Haldeman and Ehrlichman
And Jerry Ford, back then we called him 'Bozo,'
Oh, he couldn't walk and chew his gum.

Could it be that things were so much simpler then
Long before I'd given up my throne?
If I had the chance to do it all again,
Tell me, would I? WOULD I!!!

Mem-ries, how I cherish one and each,
Alger Hiss and even Checkers, as I walk along the beach,
It was the laughter that I regret most
Whenever I remember the way we were.

Just before the credits appear on the screen, the camera pans across the darkened room to David Frost, sitting in a corner, still taking notes, but now crying along with everybody else.

4. Let's All Start Talking Gooder

Safire is what closes on Saturday night.

Until I was nineteen years old and read *The Caine Mutiny*, I did not know the meaning of the word "paranoid." Today, the average 12-year-old applies the word "paranoid" to his friends with easy familiarity, as a sort of sing-song playground put-down, as in "Freddy Jones is paranoid." And the same 12-year-old has also been at ease with the word "shit" since he or she was five years old. Since, therefore, this book contains that word several times, it can be allowed in any grammar school library, and if it contained the word two times fewer than it does, it could even be allowed in any kindergarten library.

I have no doubt that in our time, this word will be legitimized into public use, joining such former no-no's as "pregnant," "abortion," and "leg." (The mid-Victorian word was "limb.") I suppose we could draw the conclusion that since ornate words like "paranoid" and vulgar words like "shit" are used by kids far earlier than their parents used them, the kids are becoming worldly sooner than we did. But I suspect that once the parents are out of hearing range, the 23-year-old teachers close the door and allow the six-year-old pupils to use that particular word as often as they wish. I guess what I'm saying is, I'm paranoid about shit.

Out of all this juvenile saltiness comes the myth held by television producers that words such as "paranoid" or "schizophrenic" should be avoided on the air because the mass audience doesn't know what they mean. Once I was taping a segment of a prime-time television show. I wanted to say that since President Carter wasn't doing very well, perhaps the job was too big for one person, and we should think about putting a schizophrenic in the White House, so that when the polls came out, at least half of him would be ahead of somebody.

Whereupon the director told me that the word schizophrenic was too intellectual and I would have to say, "schizophrenic—that's a person with a split personality." Not only does this amount to explaining the joke in the process of telling it, but children on playgrounds use the word "schizo" on each other in the same way as they use "creep" or "nerd." But a grown-up TV director opts for talking down to his audience.

"Why risk taxing their brains?" say the titans of the tube, as they spare us from hearing such erudite polysyllabic words as "erudite" and "polysyllabic."

The subject of dirty language on the air reached the Supreme Court in 1977 when someone sued a New York radio station for playing an album by the comedian George Carlin that contained the so-called seven dirty words. The Court ruled that the words could not be spoken on the public airwaves. Apparently, the justices believed that if Carlin wished to broadcast the particular piece of material under discussion, he would have to substitute his original words with "excreta," "urine," "fornicate," "vagina," etcetera.

"Etcetera," although allowed by the Court, would of course be banned by the aforementioned director since, being Latin, it is *verboten* (which is German).

The Supreme Court justices are just a regular bunch of guys doing their job, but if any one of them were to mash his thumb with a hammer, he no doubt would cry out some word other than "Excreta!" But the chances of one of them hitting his thumb with a hammer on the radio or television is remote. So I agree with their decision on the nasty words, but for a different reason. These words are offensive to be sure, not because they are obscene, but because they are so tiresome and unoriginal.

Our grandparents had some wonderful expletives that should be brought back, if for no other reason than to avoid the tedious use of the current ones. "Balderdash" is one. There is no reason why "balderdash" cannot be revived as a word to describe a falsehood, and the same goes for "horsefeathers" and "poppycock" (the Supreme Court might take partial umbrage with that one. These wonderful words ought to be liberated and should no longer be the sole property of James J. Kilpatrick).

There are still far too many very offensive words which remain on the air with regularity. (That last word is one of them.) The real obscene words, since they are usually found in commercials, are not only permitted, they are heralded—"wetness," "dirty sweatsocks," "pain and itching"—ugly words that should be banned. When I asked one of the Supreme Court justices what he thought of my opinion, he said, "pooh-pooh."

There has been an attempt by a few people to call attention to a new endangered species—not the whale or the American eagle, but the English language. Let's examine what has happened to speech in America. When you consider whom our kids regard as heroes, it's no wonder that we are quickly becoming a nation of people whose elocution is a mixture of that of a disc jockey and an athlete. It just ain't cool to be articulate—you know, you know— hey, alright, super. Take away the words "you know," "hey," "alright" and "super" from an athlete or disc jockey and he'll be speechless.

Two English words that are about to become extinct are the words "yes" and "no." They are being replaced with an expression that can be interpreted as either yes *or* no. That expression is "not really." Did you play a good game today? Not really. Did you play rotten today? Not really. This national passion for ambiguity becomes tragic when you consider the final statement of the committee investigating one of the most serious crimes in our history: "President Kennedy was *probably* shot by more than one person." The Warren Commission *was* wrong? Probably. Does anybody care? Not really.

Airline clerks are human, too—they just don't talk like it. Having spent a large and unhealthy portion of my life in airplanes and airports, the constant barrage of announcements, live and recorded, delivered in military fashion by pilots, stewardesses, clerks, and others in authority, is starting to transform me from a fairly alert human into a mindless robot. Give an airline clerk a microphone to speak into and he becomes so dehumanized and automated, he sounds like an outer space Conehead on "Saturday Night Live."

Next time you fly, listen, and you'll find that every announcement contains the same three words, "at this time"; as in, "Ladies
and gentlemen, we ask at this time that you fasten your seat belts,"
or "We ask at this time that you refrain from smoking." "At this
time" is a waste of time. It doesn't mean anything. We know they
mean put out your cigarettes now, so why don't they just say it?

Imagine an airline clerk coming home to his family after making
his announcements all day. He says, "Hi, honey, I'm home. At this
time I would like to ask, how was your day?" His wife answers,
"Don't ask. The plumber was here today and at this time I would
like to announce that we are in need of a new hot water heater and
the estimated cost at this time is three hundred dollars." Then he
says, "I'd like to announce at this time that this is a fine mess to
come home to at this time, and when will dinner be ready?" And
she answers, "Not at this time."

We seem to be well on the way to establishing words to mean the
opposite of those beginning with "in-" or "un-". To speak of a
well-mannered person as being "couth" began as a joke, but perhaps the next generation will adopt "couth" as proper usage. One
of the most puzzling words to me is "invaluable." Rather than
meaning without value, the word is used to describe something
upon which a limitless value is placed. Satirist Tom Lehrer once
used the word quite literally in a thank-you note to a friend who
had sent him a gift: "I found your present to be invaluable and
some day I hope to find it valuable."

When Chief Justice Warren Burger was of the opinion that 50
percent of the trial lawyers in America were inept and inert, could
we then assume that the other 50 percent were ept and ert?

And consider the deception of the word "deceased." Come now,
when you die you certainly are not deceased; you are ceased. To
be deceased is to come back to life again. Another word of deadly
deception is *interred*. After a person dies, he is interred. If they dig
him up, is he terred?

Whenever a president's speech writer quits or is fired, much of
Washington wonders whether he wasn't writing what he was told,
or if the president simply ignored what was written for him. Perhaps speech writers for politicians are fired because most of them

can never satisfy their bosses' hunger for the single memorable phrase that will, in an instant, guarantee him lasting fame among history's noblest statesmen.

There hasn't been a phrase in an inaugural address to top John F. Kennedy's "Ask not what your country" line in 1961. The phrase was both simple and catchy, and in all the years since, not one presidential speech writer has come up with a single line that will stick.

"I offer you a new American Revolution," said Richard Nixon in 1974. I don't know what the writer had in mind with that one, but the offer didn't take. Perhaps the reference to our nation's birth should have read, "Give me liberty or play the tapes," or "We are endowed with certain inalienable rights and among these are life, liberty, and a one million dollar advance on hardcover books not including paperback rights."

In President Carter's 1979 State of the Union address, his speech writer went for the brass ring with "I offer you a New Foundation," which, although more binding than a New Revolution, was scarcely remembered a week later, except for a few girdle jokes.

Halfway through Carter's first term in office, his entire speech writing staff resigned. It seemed at the time that the president would be relying more heavily on other writers, named Matthew, Mark, Luke, and John. Carter always had trouble with speech writers, even prior to his election in 1976. It was thought that those fellows didn't quite have the knack of writing a quotable sentence—like the guy who wrote, "Sometimes I'll never lie to you." As we know, Jimmy Carter revised it into the oft repeated line that keeps coming back to haunt him: "I'll *never* lie to you."

This dissatisfaction with inept speech writers is nothing new of course, and a number of presidents have learned the hard way that they could do a better job themselves. Harry Truman's famous phrase did not begin as "The buck stops here." No, he had to let his writer go, after the man wrote, "Herein one finds the locale of the termination of the dollar."

Years before, Barbara Fritchie had a similar experience with an incompetent scribe who wrote, "Do whatever you wish with the flag, but don't touch my hair!"

"Out of here!" cried the feisty Fritchie to her cowering secretary, as she sat down and wrote a telegram to the British: "Shoot if you will this old gray head, but spare my country's flag!" Unfortunately, Western Union, true to form, sent the message as "Shoot if you will this old gay red but spare my country's fag."

The most famous presidential inaugural phrase in history might never have been uttered had not Franklin D. Roosevelt spotted the unacceptable writing in time. Otherwise, he would have said, "If ever there was something we don't have to fear, it's that!"

Historians are certain to refer to the very first major Kennedy-Carter skirmish as the "fig-leaf assertion and the baloney response." As early as the winter of 1979, Teddy Kennedy asserted that Carter's windfall profits tax was "a fig leaf over the oil companies' profits." Carter responded that Kennedy's opinion was "baloney." A snappy comeback, no matter how you slice it.

Political rhetoric often contains references to food—pork barrel, sour grapes, mushroom cloud, pie-in-the-sky. Former Senator Hugh Scott of Pennsylvania used to talk about the leavening of the dough of high idealism into the pasta of legislation. It's an old tactic to divert us from the real problems. Except that food itself is now one of the real problems.

On another occasion, President Carter said that the oil lobbyists "would descend on Congress like a chicken on a June bug." If you consult *Webster's New World Dictionary*, you'll find that the June bug of the southern United States is defined as (are you ready?) a big eater. I broke the code and predicted that the June bugs (that's Congress in Carter's speech) would devour the fig leaf, which is the profits tax in the Kennedy speech—which meant that Congress would defeat that tax.

Once, at a White House press conference, a reporter suggested that the Carter administration was overloaded with Georgians. Why not? Kennedy had Bostonians, LBJ had Texans, and Nixon had Prussians.

Carter brought up the non-Georgians, mentioning his foreign adviser Zbginiew Brzezinski. The rumor is that Brzezinski is actually Carter's cousin from Macon and that the name is just a code. If you substitute a vowel for every consonant and vice versa, interchange every third letter, and hold it up to a mirror, you have Brzezinski's real name—Jethro Gump. His foreign accent is affected. He went to Harvard where he was greatly impressed by one of the professors, a Dr. Henry Kreplinger, Kippingler, something like that. So now you know the truth. If you wake Zbginiew Brzezinski up in the middle of the night, he talks just like Billy Carter.

As the day's headlines become more and more confusing, here is a glossary of terms often found in newspaper and television reports to help in your study of current events.

LOYALTY OATH: Taken by Democratic candidates who swear they invited President Carter to campaign for them before he went up in the polls.

TIP O'NEILL: The nickname of a bellhop in Dublin.

DOORKEEPER OF THE HOUSE: The title of a GSA official who took the door home with him.

PRIVATE BILL: Your cousin in the army.

NEPOTISM: What you get when you eat too many uncooked nepots.

SODIUM NITRITES: A consumer term. Sodium nitrites are said to contain alarming traces of bacon.

BOLSHOI: The fastest growing American ballet company.

H-BOMB: A top secret, unless you can afford *Progressive* magazine, the Madison, Wisconsin, *Press Connection*, the *Chicago Tribune*, and very soon, *Mad* magazine and tee shirts.

ODD/EVEN: A practical idea that was helpful so we're phasing it out.

METRIC: A terrible idea that's a hindrance, so we're phasing it in.

CHAPPAQUIDICK: The name of a place brought up by candidates every time they say they are not going to bring it up.

POLL: A series of questions put to someone whom neither you, nor anyone you know, has ever met.

Since my college education consists of three months at the University of Miami in Florida and 28 days at George Washington University, my formal schooling in English ended with high school. Tom Snyder and I once compared notes on his show about our respective high schools. Discovering that we each attended schools run by the Jesuit Fathers, Snyder began praising the teaching order for its obviously fine product (himself). I apparently was less than enthusiastic about the effect the Jesuit system had upon me. I had had a terrible time struggling through the classical high school curriculum, with its four years of Latin and baffling mathematics. I must have given the impression that it had been of little practical use to me because several days after the show, I received a letter from a Jesuit priest calling me an ingrate for knocking their teaching methods. I wrote back explaining that my remarks had been misinterpreted, and that my incoherence probably was due to jet lag. I further stated that I thought very highly of the Jesuits' teaching methods and that if I thought otherwise, my daughter would not be entering Georgetown University in the coming fall. (She wasn't.)

The truth is that I revere the splendid educational tradition of the Jesuits, which has been of great benefit to me and my work as a humorist, as I am about to demonstrate.

I close this salute to language with an intellectual joke told to me recently by the Reverend Patrick Sullivan, S.J., of Canisius High School in Buffalo, New York, my alma mater:

Three Indian squaws were pregnant and as the time for delivery arrived, the first one went into her teepee, sat down on a bear skin rug, and delivered a son. The second one went into her teepee, sat down on a bear skin rug, and also delivered a son. However, the third one walked into her teepee, sat down on a hippopotamus skin rug, and delivered twin boys. Moral: The sons of the squaw on the hide of the hippopotamus are equal to the sum of the sons of the squaws on the other two hides.

As I tell my kids—you can't beat a good education. Irregardless of what you might think.

5. Russell's Handy Guide to Hardball Campaigning

Dress for Success!   —MOTHER THERESA

Seeking public office? Subscribe now to my simple rules for running a successful campaign. You can astound the experts, dazzle the opposition, and win the day by applying the solid virtues of trickery, deceit, and transparent veneer.

RULE NUMBER ONE: Always have splattered mud on your shoes— then everybody will think you've just returned from the boondocks.

House Speaker Tip O'Neill once said that Jimmy Carter was thought of very highly in the "boondocks." I love Tip O'Neill, but to him the boondocks is a seat at the head table at the annual dinner held by the Friendly Sons of Saint Patrick. You see, it all depends on whose boondocks you visit. In fact, the National Association of Boondocks rated the president as having all the toughness of TV's Mister Rogers. Politicians and members of the press are always coming back to Washington saying that they have been out into the land taking America's pulse. Well, the prairies over which they roam are really airport terminals; the people they talk to are paying their lecture fees. The only boondocks they see is the landscape on the wallpaper at the local Holiday Inn.

No one will believe you are in touch with the people if you admit you haven't been out of Washington in a while. You must offer positive proof that you've been staying at one motel after another all over the country. So you let it be known that you haven't drunk from anything but a plastic cup in six months.

RULE NUMBER TWO: Learn to make those hard decisions—like whether to seek an endorsement from Alan Alda or Allen Ludden.

At what point does a presidential campaign become official? Is it when a specific number of hopefuls officially declare? No. Is it when Harold Stassen's name first appears in the paper? No. Is it when Teddy Kennedy starts getting coy? None of the above. The campaign becomes official when movie stars start endorsing candidates. In the '79–'80 campaign, when the Ronald Reagan for President committee had just been formed, the list of his supporters came out, led by Pat and Debbie Boone. (Having those two alone should have caused Howard Baker and the others to head for the showers.) Reagan also had James Cagney, Frank Sinatra (let's hear those trumpets), James Stewart, Loretta Young, and Irene Dunne. It should have been all over then. I wonder if Debbie Boone knows who Irene Dunne is? A stacked deck, if ever I saw one. It was embarrassing. John Connally, where were your celebrities? Philip Crane, who did you have? How about a Muppet? Somebody. Anybody.

Remember—on the road to victory, the stars will guide you.

RULE NUMBER THREE: Let the secret of your strength be elevator shoes.

I always figured that big John Connally would get the Republican nomination, because GOP surveys seemed to imply that what the party wanted was somebody tall. The Republicans stressed America's weaknesses, but with big John Connally, we would have peace through height. I had trouble erasing a vision of Connally as Randolph Scott holding a poker hand on a Mississippi River boat, and could hear those Republican speeches: "Four years with a Sunday school teacher in the White House is too long. Send for the high sheriff. Seize the oil fields. Fill the Iranian skies with B-52s. Call out the Marines. Bring back the draft. It's too quiet around here, so let's get back to normalcy! Nominate Big John, a credit to his party." Both of them.

RULE NUMBER FOUR: Give the press a break once in a while—with constructive profanity.

Jimmy Carter finally became a real politician in the tradition of Ulysses S. Grant, Harry Truman, and Lyndon Johnson, when asked at a dinner party what he would do if Teddy Kennedy ran against him. Mr. Carter said (and for the sake of decency we'll alter the quote a bit), "I'll whip his donkey!"

Political analysts set out trying to figure out why Carter would want to whip Kennedy's donkey. Such a mulish remark could only antagonize animal lovers everywhere. And that this particular livestock is the symbol of the party of both Kennedy and Carter only added to the confusion. Democrats, of course, will be Democrats. Lyndon Johnson once picked up his dog by the ears, but he never whipped anybody's donkey. I believe that with Jimmy Carter, the whipping of the donkey symbolized the show of strength the Republicans had been clamoring for. This was not a Sunday school teacher talking. This was our commander-in-chief. And as far as Teddy was concerned, it was *his* donkey.

RULE NUMBER FIVE: Dull is beautiful.

A skillful politician can cope with insulting adjectives thrown at him by his opponents, such as crooked, loathsome, conniving, lecherous, sniveling, and liberal; these charges merely bounce off the seasoned pro. But call him dull and chances are it will hurt him badly. It happened when word got out that Senator "Scoop" Jackson once gave a fireside chat and the fire went out. Any candidate burdened with a dull label might as well go back to his floor polisher rental business.

It doesn't seem fair, because it is possible that a dull candidate can bring out the best in the voters. Here is what I mean: Let's say a candidate has all the ebullience and dash of the actor E. G. Marshall. A voter watching him long enough begins to feel like Burt Reynolds by comparison; even if he sells shelf paper at Woolworth's, he soon develops into a swashbuckler.

Let me address the voter for a moment. A dull candidate speaking at a political banquet can make you yearn to hear the clergyman's opening prayer all over again. The discovery that you had more religion than you thought can make you feel better. If there are many dull candidates in an election, you may be driven to seek new horizons. Engulfed by dullness, you may wish to get away from those boring monotones and flee to someplace more exciting, like Greenland. Or in the words of one poor voter, "If I have to listen to one more speech by Jerry Ford, I'm going to Winnipeg for some action."

Attention dull candidates: Be proud of your dullness. As William McKinley once said, "If you've got it, flaunt it." You might start by beginning every speech with a knock-knock joke. Drab is good. Otherwise, Millard Fillmore, Chester Alan Arthur, Rutherford B. Hayes, and Martin Van Buren would have bored in vain.

RULE NUMBER SIX: Don't be afraid to spend a lot of money advertising your mediocrity.

Eighty-five percent of those winning the race for the United States Senate did so by spending more than their opponents. This means that it is still okay to have been born in a log cabin as long as the cabin was in the right neighborhood. The Senate is a rich man's club and the successful politician freely admits it: "Ah yes. I was born in a log cabin—Mother and Father were on a rustic holiday at the time."

Since it's mostly the rich who can win elections, this brings about a whole new style of campaign rhetoric: "Let's look at the record. I've got six one-minute commercials a day on radio and television while my opponent hands out his lousy balloons."

As a big spender, your campaign speeches should leave no doubt in the voter's mind that your impoverished opponent hasn't got a dime. "I deserve to win because I'm not afraid to tell it like it is. I've spent a half million clams on TV alone! Let's see my opponent top that. He's a loser, that's what he is—look at his old car and that baggy suit—he hasn't got a

chance. Let's examine his commercials. They're a disgrace—
no violins, no sunsets. Is that the kind of man you want in
Washington? I should think not!"

RULE NUMBER SEVEN: Declare yourself the winner two minutes
after the polls open.

Every election year, the networks declare the winner earlier
and earlier. I remember in the Wisconsin primary in 1976, the
experts at ABC declared Morris Udall to be the winner when
he was only leading by 7/10 of a percentage point. They have
since corrected this immature forecasting, and they now wait
until a candidate is ahead by 8/10 of a percentage point. How
would ABC like it if the Nielsen rating service stopped two
winos on the street and asked them if they watched "The
Love Boat"?

Prior to the 1980 Iowa caucuses, they heralded the
projection that the next leader of the free world would be
chosen by three waitresses and the owner of a hardware store
in Cedar Rapids. Why this rush to name the winner before
the votes are in? These people count their chickens before the
rooster and the hen even go on the honeymoon. Long before
the voters go to the polls in Alaska and Hawaii, the networks
in New York tell them which lever they are going to pull.

I have a suggestion. This may seem crazy and far out, but
it's time for drastic measures. Wait until everyone votes, then
count the ballots. I tell you, it can be done; they do it at race-
tracks all the time and without network projections. Which-
ever horse gallops across the finish line ahead of the other
horses is the winner!

RULE NUMBER EIGHT: While campaigning in an ethnic neighborhood, the bowling shirt is never worn with a tie.

Reporters covering political campaigns, particularly in the
northern industrial cities, by tradition trek their equipment
into the ethnic neighborhood bars every four years in order to
ascertain the mood of the area. It's a wonder more of them
don't get punched in the nose as they sidle up to a patron and
say, "Pardon me, sir, I gather by your appearance that you are

a member of this nation's great working class. I wonder if you could share your thoughts on how George Bush's domestic policies interface with the citizenry here in Pittsburgh?" Just once I'd like to see some burly welder stick the reporter's microphone into his pitcher of Miller's.

The candidates also make a beeline from the airport to the nearest blue-collar hangout for a crash course on the "ethnic milieu," as if to say, "Give me one Pulaski Day parade and two beers with a pinball player in Scranton, and I'll have my finger on the pulse of Eastern Europe."

"—and so, here at Helminiak's Tap Room of Akron, Ohio, you might say, Walter, that the people are suspicious of any candidate until he buys a round for the house. Bob Shieffer, CBS News, Akron. That's the way it is. When you're out of Schlitz, you're out of wisdom."

What these political geniuses don't seem to know is that the old stereotypes are not reliable and that Poles, Italians, Croations, Czecho-Serbians, Litho-Hungarian-Slavo-Buffalonians, etcetera, etcetera, also go to libraries. If you're an ethnic, when an election year rolls around and you wish to avoid all the hoards of reporters, photographers, technicians, columnists, and candidates, go to a museum; they'll never look for you there.

I've had a lot of fun over the years with a story that I originally made up about Sargent Shriver during his several brief tries for political office. The story can be applied to others— perhaps a George Bush or any office seeker not appearing to be completely at home in the atmosphere of a blue-collar saloon. We first see the candidate performing the ritual of shaking hands in front of a steel mill with the workers as they pass through the gate coming off the day shift. Our hero, wearing a hard hat with his suit, arm extended, sings out his salutation, "Hi, there, I'm Sargent Shriver, and I'd appreciate your vote." Half ignoring him, the steel workers hurriedly make their way to the gin mill across the street from the main gate of the plant. The candidate, undaunted, follows the men over and enters the place. As Kenny Rogers whines "Lucille" over the juke box in a duet with the electronic bonging of the pinballs, the neon Anheuser-Busch eagle over the bar illuminates the "No Checks Cashed" sign, and the 30-year-old scent of thousands of tapped kegs fills the air, the candidate joins in the fun. He bellies up to the bar and says, "I'll have a Courvoisier, please." The room falls silent and the bartender says, "Do you want mustard on it?"

6. I Brake for Lawyers

Shucks, I'm just a plain old country lawyer, comprendez-vous?   —ANON

It's not that I don't like lawyers, it's just that there are so many of them. We who dwell in the nation's capital have learned to live side by side with those of the legal profession, and we do so out of necessity, for Washington without lawyers would be like Rome without priests. Remove the lawyers from Washington and the city would become a silent movie set inhabited by just a few people including nonlawyers Jimmy Carter and myself.

There are tax attorneys, constitutional attorneys, patent attorneys, trial lawyers, criminal lawyers, and lawyer-criminals. The town is infested with legal clerks, legal secretaries, legislative aides, legislative assistants and assistant legislative aides. Even the owner of the football team is a lawyer. They make up a multidivisioned army in pinstripes—the Brooks Brothers Brigade—and if all of those pinstripes were extended horizontally, they would encircle the globe several times. The poor animals who unwillingly gave their hides to be turned into legal attaché cases carried in Washington is something I'd rather not think about.

This massive legal presence is unavoidable in the place where our laws are made, interpreted, enforced, and sometimes broken, all by the same people. Whenever a bar association convenes, the assemblage always observes a moment of silence, for their dear departed brothers now serving in minimum security prisons. It is usually a prayer for those who are doing three years at hard tennis.

One of the hottest categories on the lecture circuit is the law-yer-felon-author. Lawyer-felon-authors command handsome fees for making speeches, certainly much more than mere lawyers or even lawyer-authors. I advise anyone wishing to get into the public speaking biz to commit a crime, get caught, be convicted, and do some time in the pokey. When you are released, you can add an extra thousand dollars to your lecture fee.

A visitor to a prison today is likely to see signs posted around the compound saying, "You are all invited to a Meet-the-Author autograph party this afternoon in Cell Block 3." Because of the large number of authors-in-residence throughout our correctional institutions, outside work programs must be revamped to allow the prisoner ample time for guest appearances on the "Today" show, "Good Morning, America," and the Dick Cavett Show.

In an all-out effort to reform our penal system, some of the improvements afforded the modern inmate include better food, more recreation, and a higher percentage of the paperback income. This heightened focus on the lawyer-felon-author came about when some of the participants in the Watergate mess wrote books while incarcerated. These included such works as *The Ends of Power*, by H. R. Haldeman, and *The Company*, by John Ehrlichman. The latter was made into a TV drama; however, the author could not watch the show because it was on after lights out. These works sold very well and were probably the most famous books written in prison since *Mein Kampf*.

I suppose I should have been a lawyer. I would have fit in better in my adopted city if I had. I even tried faking it a few times on airplanes when the inevitable question arises in the conversation with the person seated next to me: "Where are you from?"

"Washington."

"Oh, you a lawyer?"

"Uh, yeah."

"So am I."

"Oh, well, uh, I'm really a comedian."

"That's not funny. You don't look like a comedian. Are you sure you are not a lawyer?"

"No."

It is not my intention here to take swipes at all lawyers but to

cite some of the laws we all must deal with. The only letter to the
editor I ever wrote in my life was to the *Washington Post* to ridicule the enforcement of the "blue" law in Virginia. A grocer in
that state had been arrested for selling two grapefruits on a Sunday, which was against the archaic law; as was walking your goat
or double parking your mule on the Sabbath. I wrote:

> Regarding the apprehension of a grocer for selling
> grapefruit on Sunday, thank God they stopped that
> man in time. Where once this evil yellow fruit was only
> used by jazz musicians and aimless drifters of the lost
> generation, today grapefruit has found its way, not only
> into high schools, but grammar schools as well! Now
> that that monster is safely put away, they ought to
> throw away the key so that he and all the perverted gro-
> cers can no longer corrupt society with the yellow
> peril—grapefruit!

We're all familiar with that dubious tax law that bestows a higher
tax rate upon a husband and wife with separate incomes and a
lower rate upon an unmarried couple living together. There have
been publicized cases of married people who at the end of the year
go down to the Caribbean and get a quickie divorce (as opposed to
a longie divorce) that is retroactive for the whole previous year.
They take a vacation on the tax savings and then remarry after
January 1.

There is at least one couple who has been doing this for years.
Each time they get married to each other, instead of saying, "I do,"
they say, "Don't I always?" By repeating the marriage ceremony
so often, they not only have saved thousands in taxes, but they
now have 37 chafing dishes. Every time they get married, the or-
ganist plays "Love for Sale," and I suspect that their favorite
movie is *Same Time, Next Year*. After one of the couple's mar-
riages, authorities became suspicious when the couple ran hugging
and kissing under a shower of flying rice to their car parked in
front of the divorce court.

Unless this law is changed—and quickly—more and more cou-
ples will learn the combination to this revolving door wedlock.

And as the Treasury loses, we'll need a windfall profits tax. Not to build a transportation system, but to support the bartenders and surfing instructors of the Dominican Republic and Haiti.

When Jimmy Carter first came on the scene around 1975, one of the most appealing things about him was that he was not a lawyer. His "Vote for me, I'm not a lawyer," had a refreshing ring to it. Comedian Lenny Bruce's overly candid political character of twenty years ago said, "Elect me, I'm not a nut!" In the reign of Richard Nixon, the declaration became "I am not a crook."

So what's next? Why didn't any of Carter's opponents say, "Elect me, I'm not a peanut farmer/nuclear engineer?" No doubt, in our time, a candidate will mount the stump to proclaim, "Elect me, I am not a man."

The nonlawyer halo becomes tarnished a bit, however, when we look at the handful of presidents who entered the White House from outside the legal profession. They include those two paragons of virtue, Ulysses S. Grant and Warren G. Harding.

At one of his low points in the polls, Carter, in an effort to revive his populist appeal, picked a target that most presidents could not zero in on—lawyers. He had already attacked doctors, and after his attack on lawyers, people began wondering if Indian chiefs would be next. "The lawyers of this country constitute a hierarchy of privilege," cried Carter. Bert Lance later said to him, "Leave me out of this."

White-collar crime was on the rise (thousands of white collars are stolen annually) and Carter blamed the lawyers. This is what is known, in Ralph Nader's words, as "crime in the suites." Carter's disregard for lawyers raised questions about his future appointments, giving rise to the speculation that perhaps some future Supreme Court justice would be an electrician.

There has been a growing interest in legal circles in permitting lawyers to specialize in the same manner as doctors, and to grant licenses accordingly, which is all we need. If you're charged with stealing a horse and a pig, you'll need two lawyers, one specializing in pigs and one specializing in horses.

Imagine what specialization would do to property settlements in divorce cases. The husband tells his lawyer he wants the color TV and the coffee table, and the lawyer tells him he doesn't handle

furniture. (Neither does the wife's lawyer. He probably special-
izes in boats, cars, and jewelry).

Under lawyer-specialization, the famous Scopes "Monkey
Trial" would have been much more complicated. Clarence Dar-
row probably wouldn't have been allowed to handle the case, since
monkeys must be covered by an environmental specialist.

We are living in the age of alternatives—alternative lifestyles, alternative approaches, alternative publications, and more and more
judges are handing out what lawyers are calling alternative sentences. Instead of receiving a jail term, a defendant might be ordered to do penance in some way directly connected with his of-
fense. For example, a drunk driver might be sentenced to attend
Alcoholics Anonymous meetings. Or a slum landlord might be
sentenced to a year in one of his own dumps.

Supposing they had had alternate sentencing at the time of some
of history's great criminals. What might the sentences have been?

"Blackbeard, you have been a terror on the high seas for too
long. I hereby sentence you to four years in the United States
Navy."

"Al Capone, the law has finally caught up with you. I sentence
you to write a two-thousand-word essay on why Chicago is the
most peaceful city in the world."

"Marie Antoinette, this time you've gone too far. Let 'em eat
cake, eh? Let's see if you can slim down on nothing but hardtack
and gruel."

"King George the Third, you tyrant, you—ten years picking
tobacco in Virginia ought to change your ways."

"That dastardly sneak attack on Pearl Harbor was too much,
Hirohito. Your sentence is to spend the war as a bellhop at the
Royal Hawaiian Hotel."

Whenever a student of the law wishes to do any research on
libel, he or she is wise to consult a humorist, since we are usually
the ones who commit libel. At least, it is implied that we do. I'm
always asked such questions as "Have you ever been sued?" or
"Do the people you joke about ever get mad?" (God, I hope so.)

Let us first look up the word "libel" in the dictionary. Ah, here
it is—just before "liberal."

Libel: 1. Any written or printed statement, or any sign, picture, etc., tending to injure a person's reputation unjustly. [Unjustly—there's a handy loophole.] 2. The act or crime of publishing such a thing. [Make up your mind, Webster; what do you mean, "act" *or* "crime"? Is it a crime or isn't it? I caught your act last night and it was a crime.] 3. Anything that gives an unflattering picture of the subject with which it is dealing. [This dictionary is beginning to sound totalitarian. Unflattering? I should have been arrested years ago.]

My own personal definition of libel is: if the guy didn't do it and you said he did it, and you didn't get a laugh when you said it, it's libel. If I say, "Senator Bribewell spent two weeks in Acapulco last January as the guest of the Consolidated Frisbee Corporation, and then came back to Washington and voted for the defense appropriation bill to provide the Army with 8 million frisbees," that would probably be libelous, providing the senator did no such thing, of course. Since it is a flat-out statement, it is not funny. But what if his real name was Bidewell or Slidewell and I changed it to "Bribewell"? Or, I might say, "I went to visit the senator last January in his private office—a cabana in Acapulco. As he greeted me, he stood up, dropped his wallet, and broke his foot."

No two lawyers will agree on what is libel and what isn't, and I suspect that attorneys employed by the radio and television networks spend a great deal of their days flipping coins. Shortly after I began doing a daily radio commentary for NBC, I taped a piece that never got on the air. It was at the time President Carter had to fire his White House expert on drug problems, Dr. Peter Bourne, who had been accused of falsifying a prescription. The story was ballyhooed for about a week—a medium-sized scandal during which I recorded that there was a rumor in Washington that when Dr. Bourne was in the White House, he often wrote highly classified, top-secret prescriptions. As secret documents are stamped "For the President's Eyes Only," these prescriptions were labeled, "For the President's Nose Only."

The line never went out over the air, and frankly I knew that NBC would censor it. But having just begun the series, I wanted to test the system. After recording the Dr. Bourne piece on the telephone over a direct line to New York, I hung up and sat there waiting for the phone to ring. I waited for about 60 seconds. The call came from NBC in New York, which is in the RCA Building, situated at the vortex of global media power. The call came from the producer, whose voice was wavering between hysteria and incoherence: "I am sitting here with *three* NBC lawyers and we are all in *full* agreement that that routine you just sent up here is in very bad taste." I said, "For that you need lawyers? I *know* it's in bad taste."

"Taste," unlike "libel," is not a legal term.

"Hey, buddy, what are ya in for?"

"Bad taste."

"Get away from me, ya creep."

A few months later, dat ol' debbil Censor came around again. This time I suggested over the air that, inasmuch as there had been an official pardon of Richard Nixon, we as a people should show equal charity and forgive the Pinto. I further suggested that, really, the only thing wrong with the car was the name—Pinto. It was a puny sounding name and nobody wanted to drive anything with a runty, sawed-off name like that. I advised the Ford Motor Company to show a little imagination in their advertising and give this beleagured car a more majestic name, such as "The New Ford Hindenburg."

> COMMERCIAL: "Yes, with the new Ford Hindenburg, we've enlarged the gas tank, filled it with helium, and placed it on top of the car. Think of the fun you'll have when you say to the parking attendant, 'It's the gray blimp with the white mud flaps.' "

Ford needn't have been concerned about that routine. NBC had a better idea. The objection was that because Ford was steeped in litigation over several crashes involving Pintos, the idea of associating the automobile with a known, historical dirigible explosion was absolutely prohibitive. Of course, I had no idea what they were talking about. I was thinking of General von Hindenburg, the World War I military leader who used to get 27 on the highway and 18 in town. So you see, one man's libel is another man's blimp.

The possibility of legal action can be avoided by the use of the word "allegedly." On the day that the alleged Carmine Galante was allegedly blown away by six alleged persons wearing alleged ski masks in an alleged Italian restaurant in alleged Brooklyn—on that same day, the Pope in Rome reaffirmed the traditional doctrine of Heaven, Hell, and eternal damnation. A few days later, the archbishop of New York City refused to give Mr. Galante a Catholic funeral because he said he wanted to avoid a scandal, and not out of judgment of Mr. Galante's soul or his intimate relationship with God. So the question is where is Carmine Galante—Heaven, Hell, or some cosmic detention center with Al Capone, Lucky Luciano, and Baby Face Nelson?

When the press reported that six men wearing ski masks shot Mr. Galante as he was eating in an Italian restaurant in Brooklyn while smoking a cigar, it's a wonder that there wasn't a protest against the media by the Cigar-Smoking Italian Skiers Anti-Defamation League. The killers must have been imposters since everyone knows that it was off-season at every ski resort in Brooklyn. Once again, the press blew the whole thing out of proportion. Actually, Mr. Galante (whose real name is Lars Smorgasbord) choked on a chicken bone at a Methodist Church supper in Cedar Rapids, Iowa.

Traveling through the Midwest several years ago, I picked up a newspaper and saw a headline on the front page that read, "Supreme Court Considers Homosexuality." My initial reaction was, *all nine?* The legal and political aspects of homosexuality have entered into various ballotings across the country. Californians once voted on a proposal that said, "Check yes or no. Do you agree if you have homosexual teachers you will automatically have homosexual students, since teachers are role models, and if they are homosexual their students will grow up to be the same?" After giving this a great deal of thought, I decided that if that were true, today I would be a nun.

I have an occasional fantasy during which I imagine myself to be the tenth Supreme Court justice handing down decisions right along there with the other nine. I have often sided with the minority on some of the high court's big rulings, and one of those times was in regard to the decision on unannounced searches.

The Court upheld a decision allowing the police to make unannounced searches of homes or offices occupied by persons innocent of any crimes. Yes, friends, organized crime marches on, but you'd better hide the family album. As the police may now rummage through the belongings of the innocent, we can assume the Justice Department will set up a Diary and Love Letter Division. A love letter clerk could call a particular paragraph to your attention: "Now when you wrote, 'My dearest darling, I'm counting the days until I can gaze into your limpid blue eyes and kiss your ruby red lips,' what were you trying to hide?"

The Diary clerk could keep as evidence such lurid accounts as, "Dear Diary, today we went to Disneyland and saw a big rocket ship."

Because of the ruling of the Supreme Court, police departments could create an inspector in charge of wallet snapshots and family photographs. Newspapers were hit the hardest by the decision, because their offices now may be indiscriminately searched. In which case, the front page may one day bear a government stamp of approval, just like a side of beef.

There's no doubt that if this decision had been in effect earlier, Richard Nixon would have served two full terms, and after that, every knee would have bent in homage to His Supreme Highness, Spiro Agnew.

In a later ruling when I again voted with the losers, the Supreme Court allowed that a judge could order a reporter, charged with libel, to describe his state of mind at the time he wrote a particular story. After that decision, it would have been a wonderful touch in community relations if the telephone operators at the Supreme Court answered the phone by saying, "Good morning, Supreme Court. Penny for your thoughts."

I became afraid of my own shadow after that decision was handed down. Libel again. Theoretically, if they can peek into the state of mind of a reporter, they can do it to your average political comedian.

This led me to do a piece on NBC's "Real People" (their censors are a bit looser than radio's) in front of the Court itself in Washington. The theme was, Are Supreme Court justices real people? You be the judge. I said, "In light of a recent Supreme Court decision, before I comment on it, let me take a precaution which, because of that decision, is now necessary. I had better de-

scribe to you my state of mind. I feel fine today, even though six
justices voted in favor of exploration into the state of mind of jour-
nalists charged with libel. Let me say that I feel no malice toward
those justices, even though they are a bunch of silly old ninnies.
My state of mind is that I am not being malicious by calling them
silly old ninnies. I love and respect the Supreme Court, and I love
and respect the silly old ninnies who work there. The justices can
sue me for libel if they wish. My state of mind is good; so they can
peek inside my brain if they so desire—but they'll have to pay for
the hypnotist. Well, that's my commentary. Let them do with me
what they will. However, one thing bothers me. Am I going to
have to go through this every day?"

Thirty-five-year-old Allan Bakke entered into the legal journals
for all time, along with Dred Scott and Mallory, after he was
turned down for entrance at the Medical School of the University
of California at Davis because of the school's affirmative action
policy. I voted with my fellow justices in support of Bakke. As I
understood it, he would be allowed to enter the medical school so
long as affirmative action would be adhered to. In other words,
when he became a doctor, 16 percent of his patients would have to
be Lithuanian/Chicano women who were born in North Dakota.

The day of the Bakke decision was an enormous legal event,
with one of the largest crowds in Supreme Court history gathered
in front of the building. The media had been giving the story enormous play as a sort of legislative Super Bowl. The big event
pleaded for Howard Cosell's cogent appraisal: "The scrappy, but
aging future practitioner of the Hippocratic art emerged with the
blessings of the robed jurists in a heated five to four marathon. . . ."

The Supreme Court may have cleared the way for Bakke to get
his M.D., but the media had already bestowed upon him a C.D.—
celebrity doctor.

I turn for the last time to the subject of libel. We're all familiar
with that little disclaimer that can still be found at the beginning of
a novel. The disclaimer is: "The characters in this story are fictitious, and any resemblance to actual persons living or dead is
purely coincidental." In December of 1979, I once again found
myself on the losing end of the bench when the Court refused to
review a case in which a man sued an author for libel, and won,
because he thought that a fictitious character in a book the author

had written, resembled him. Naturally, nobody would sue if he resembled a fictitious character portrayed in a book as being a fine, upstanding, and stalwart fellow. However, in this case, the character was a slimy and oafish no-account. The real-life person who sued (whose name we'd better not bother about here) must have been a slimy and oafish no-account himself; otherwise, how else could he resemble the book character?

The plaintiff was awarded 75 thousand dollars in the suit, so he obviously figured it was worth the money to publicly admit that he was indeed slimy. But by deciding not even to review the case, the Supreme Court let the suit stand, which, I believe, shoots down *that* little disclaimer.

Doesn't a ruling like this set a precedent that could discourage any fledgling writers of fiction from even bothering? This seemingly silly decision on the part of the Court doesn't even allow for the common sense notion of coincidence.

It isn't difficult to imagine what a law suit such as this could have done to the authors of some of the classics. If, for example, *Moby Dick* were written today, Ralph Nader could sue on the grounds that the giant whale symbolizes a huge corporation such as General Motors, and Captain Ahab was really Ralph Nader. Or "Little Red Riding Hood"—an unflattering portrayal of the big, bad wolf dressed up like Grandma? What would have the world's transvestites done with that one? There can be no doubt that the pesticide manufacturers would not have stood for the idea of Snow White almost dying from that poison apple. The list goes on—how about Hansel and Gretel? Two lost children running toward the gingerbread house? I can hear Jerry Brown and Linda Ronstadt calling their attorneys now.

Yes, the Supreme Court has opened up a can of real, not fictitious, worms, not to mention a few poison apples. Incidentally, the characters in the previous paragraph were fictitious and any resemblance to actual persons living or dead is probably libelous.

The Brethren, by Bob Woodward and Scott Armstrong, is an unflattering portrayal of the highest court in the land. When it came out, the justices, unlike the rest of us mere mortals, could steal away to their chambers and hide from the criticism.

Chief Justice Warren Burger remained unflustered by *The Brethren*, which pictured him as being terribly formal and pompous. Whether it was an accurate portrayal, I don't know, although I heard that when he read the book, he became so shaken that his powdered wig fell off.

Chief Burger, or as he is listed in the phone book, Burger, Chief, once invited me to provide the after-dinner entertainment at an annual banquet that takes place in the private dining room of the Supreme Court building. Flattered, my immediate reaction to the invitation was that I could boast to my friends in the entertainment world that, in the parlance of show biz, I was going to play a "class room." The only other "room" higher in status than the Supreme Court private dining room, I suppose, would be the White House itself. My ego blowing up uncontrollably, I imagined how I would casually drop into future conversations that "I have played the Court." My Las Vegas-oriented colleagues in comedy may point out that well, after all, the dining room is not the "big room" but only the lounge, but I would pay them no mind. What did they want me to do—tell Burger that I would only work the Supreme Court chamber?

The big night arrived. The guest list was a Who's Who of the nation's judiciary—federal judges, senior partners of blue chip law firms, plus a sprinkling of corporate heads. You get the picture—everybody had carfare to get home.

Our chief justice fancies himself a gourmet, and the dinner itself was a hymn to culinary splendor, including a few dishes prepared by our host himself. Dish after dish arrived accompanied by an impeccable selection of the world's noblest wines.

I enjoyed none of it. Under other circumstances, I would have reveled in such haute cuisine, but knowing I had to perform immediately after the dinner made for considerable apprehension, which was compounded by the fact that Warren Burger paid me the honor of seating me immediately to his right. While I did my best to hold up my end of the conversation ("I just dreaded the Dred Scott decision"), the tension I felt exceeded my normal pre-show jitters, perhaps because of a premonition of what was about to happen. At the same time, Burger was in a highly jovial mood, exuding charm, holding court more like a chief host than a chief justice.

At last the moment arrived. Chief Justice Burger rose and the

---

AND THAT REMINDS ME . . .

Just you wait! We'll all buy woodburning stoves, and they'll raise the price of trees.

It's been suggested that President Carter wants a tax credit for the use of woodburning stoves in order to please New Hampshire where, in addition to such stoves, they have important primaries. Why do we only hear about tax incentives in relation to heating and none concerning air-conditioning? Wooden stoves aren't too numerous in sunny Florida, which also has an important primary, so, how about a credit for purchases of blocks of ice? Regarding woodburning stoves, I've looked in every appliance store in town, and darn if I can find one. The President's message inspired me to be a pioneer. Go out and chop wood every morning, and carry it up the elevator to my condominium, and throw it into the woodstove. So, this challenge must be met by the appliance companies. I envision General Electric, under their new subsidiary General Kindling, coming out with the latest in woodburning comfort— the all-cast Ben Franklin Model for cooking and heating the patriotic way. Just set the automatic timer—one log for medium rare, two logs for well done, and as long as Jimmy Carter is installing a solar system in the White House, he might as well set an example and put in a woodburning stove. Then he can deliver a fireside chat from the kitchen.

---

room fell silent as he proposed a toast "to the President of the United States."

"To the President of the United States" we intoned, and I would swear I could hear a heel click. He then proceeded to introduce "the evening's entertainment" with an introduction no one could live up to. It might better have been applied to Arturo Toscanini or Sir Lawrence Olivier.

The opening joke of a humorous monologue determines the success or failure of the following 30 or 40 minutes. Some performers have a style of beginning very slowly, not minding a few moments of silence, and then gradually building to their stronger material. I cannot do that. I have to score within the first minute; otherwise I lose all confidence in what I have prepared. If joke A doesn't work, then neither will joke B, C, D, or E. What caused the disaster that followed was entirely my fault. The choice of joke A in this case was, shall we say, in questionable taste. I said, "Good evening, I want to thank the Chief Justice for inviting me here, which, in my mind, was the only decision he ever made which made any sense."

This brash impudence might have worked a little later in the show, after I had endeared myself to the audience, but to begin by a jab at the host in this particular setting was unwise. I say unwise because the only sound to be heard after I delivered the line was the gentle whir of the air conditioning.

Onward I plunged and came to the sure-fire stuff, but they would have none of it. Punching, jabbing, let's go to a song, body language, dialects—all was in vain. It was like swimming through glue. I now knew the meaning of "sober as a judge." The wine might as well have been Gatorade. Burger looked like he was in severe pain, as if he had just learned that Jane Fonda had been appointed to the bench. It wasn't working and everybody knew it, but I continued. The audience looked as amused as the oil paintings of Oliver Wendell Holmes and John Marshall peering down on the assemblage. My all-consuming desire at the moment was to get off, gracefully if possible, just to be somewhere else, anyplace, Devil's Island, Leavenworth, who cared? My pulse was a trip hammer, my throat the Mojave Desert. By now, my timing and delivery were completely gone. The main activity of the men consisted of looking at their watches. Finally, The End. I sang the last note of the final song, and, would you believe it, there was applause—applause of gratitude and thanksgiving that it was over for yes, we had all suffered together. I awaited sentencing from literally the highest court in the land.

It has taken me months before I could write this down. The pain is still there, and even now, the hand trembles as I relive those awful moments. We can learn from our personal Hiroshimas, and one lesson is that sometimes working a "class room" isn't worth the pain.

Another lesson is that you can't be funny in church.

7. Lost in the Sports Department

Sic Semper Adidas
(We'll never run out of sneakers)

There are grown men who wear knee-high athletic socks on weekends and have never played a sport in their lives. Poll takers conclude that Muhammed Ali is the most popular human. No president, no pope, no humanitarian will ever be as loved as Babe Ruth. Men and women who "play" for a living are envied by those who work for a living. My problem is that I haven't owned a pair of sneakers since I was nine.

It took courage on my part to make a confession like that. Do you know anyone who doesn't own a pair? Dapper septuagenarians in double-breasted suits and boutonnieres can be seen strolling in the same style of sneakers worn by their great-grandchildren. Everyone wears the footwear of the super jocks.

Except me. It's not that I have no appreciation of the skills and rigors of athletic competition. I have. But year after year I'm the one watching the movie on the odd channel during the Super Bowl game.

I've never confessed these aberrations to anyone, and even as I write them, a feeling of being unclean comes over me and I feel guilty and ashamed by my all-too-casual interest in sports. Therefore, I have at times created certain deceptions to give the impression that I fit in. One of these is a step-by-step program to trick people into thinking I am a golfer even though my lifetime average on the links (three games) is 146. This program is particularly useful to the nongolfer in the spring, when the guys at the office can talk of little else.

STEP ONE: Let the neighbors see you sitting in front of your house wiping off your clubs. If the guy next door invites you to play, tell him you want to rest your sore back a few days.

STEP TWO: Constantly practice your nonexistent golf swing—in crowded elevators, supermarket checkout lines, and so on.

STEP THREE: Sleep with your golf bag. This may affect your marriage, but then golf always does.

STEP FOUR: Leave loose tees lying all over the place—your car, desk, medicine cabinet, and falling out of your pants' pockets.

STEP FIVE: Golf shoes are pretty snazzy looking off the course as well. Your wife may not appreciate the tiny potholes in the kitchen linoleum, but she should have thought of that before she married a star athlete.

STEP SIX: Every man looks good in one of those jaunty golf hats. Try and get one from a prestige country club and, of course, wear it in the office.

STEP SEVEN: Sit under a sun lamp too long and burn your face. Then tell your friends about the 54 holes you played last Tuesday—in Brazil.

STEP EIGHT: In order to be convincing as a terrific golfer, the game must dominate your conversations. You must ask every person you meet "How ya hittin' 'em?"

Good luck on your nongame, though you won't really need it. Your scores will always be fantastic.

There is a certain type of golfer who, while a proficient player, always lets his opponent win. This kind of golfer is called a lobbyist. Since lobbyists only play golf with senators and congressmen or presidents, they must always lose. Nobody ever has seen a lobbyist win a golf game unless he's playing with another lobbyist. However, two lobbyists playing golf can only mean one thing—the politician didn't show up. When it comes to throwing the game, some lobbyists can be less than subtle about it, as in the case of the fellow who, when playing with a senator, always teed off with his putter.

Several dramatic crises in sports concerned Pope John Paul I and his successor John Paul II. One of the networks preempted a scheduled pro football game in favor of broadcasting the coronation of Pope John Paul I, live from Rome. Naturally, the switchboards at the local stations across the country were jammed by irate fans calling to complain that the coronation of the pope was interfering with their religion.

It's downright suicidal for television's decision-makers to tamper with the will of the faithful who worship at the Shrine of the Inflated Pigskin. I don't doubt that it crossed their minds at the network that day to see if the pope couldn't at least read a few scores during his sermon.

Like all the other religions, the Church of the Holy Football has many colorful rituals. During the service (game) the worshipers act out a rite of jumping up and down, drinking a liquid from a ceremonial flask, and chanting the words "Charge," "Dee-fence," and "Boo."

The faithful at the Shrine are steadfast in their Sunday devotion, which is always followed by the traditional Monday argument (or wars of religion) around the office water cooler. This body of water is not to be confused with the office pool, which is made of paper. This paper, partaken by the devoted ones, renders them cleansed of their money.

The highest of their holy days is called Super Bowl Sunday. It is, of course, televised, and let us pray that it will never fall on the day of the coronation of a pope, because if it does, the networks will be faced with a hell of a decision.

A similar decision came, in fact, in 1979, when John Paul II, visiting the United States, was scheduled to say a mass before an estimated one million people on the mall in Washington. This was on an autumn Sunday afternoon when the Redskins were playing on the otherside of town. Along with dire predictions of horrendous traffic and crowd congestion came the idea that some of the confusion could be eliminated by the pope's saying mass at the stadium during half-time.

Occasionally the gods smile upon the Washington Redskins

when they have a good reason. When this happens, the coach be-comes a more prominent celebrity than the president. George Allen enjoyed such esteem for years until, like some presidents, he argued with his employers and was canned. Allen returned to his native California, went to San Clemente, knocked on the door, and said, "Got room for one more?"

A man can sense when the axe is about to fall. George Allen be-came suspicious when he went to his office at the Redskins' train-ing camp and found his desk in the end zone and his contract in the whirlpool. Allen's personality was completely the opposite of that of the team's owner, the famous attorney Edward Bennett Wil-liams. Allen's rather straightlaced manner is in contrast to Wil-liams's, which is, to say the least, more garrulous.

The coach had been complaining that Williams had a habit of calling him on the phone in the middle of the night suggesting plays and advising him on which quarterback to use. For all any-one knows, the phone calls could have been made at 9:30 P.M. George wasn't exactly a swinger. I observed him at the Shoreham Hotel on New Year's Eve a few years ago and he really let himself go with reckless abandon. At the stroke of midnight he had not one but *two* marshmallows in his cocoa.

I don't know what the future holds for the Redskins, but George Allen gave Washington some great seasons, getting more out of old men than Zsa Zsa Gabor.

I don't discuss sports on my shows a great deal, but here is a radio speech I delivered on June 7, 1978, using a slight Franklin D. Roosevelt delivery. The night before the show, the Washington Bullets had defeated the Seattle Supersonics for the world basket-ball championship. Here's the speech:

> Yesterday—June the seventh, a day that will live in in-famy—the enemies of Washington having launched a provoked attack were forced to capitulate behind their own lines. With a slaughter that showed the world that the recent posture of toughness in Washington was au-thentic, all of its potential enemies were put on notice that this capital city was one to be reckoned with. Merely hours after President Carter bared his teeth and informed the world that we were in no mood to be

pushed around, we struck with a might that gave credence to the president's warning.

And this morning, the dastardly foes of Washington who dared to think, as recently as yesterday, that they could mount an offensive against us, woke up to a city in shambles. And how long it will take Seattle to recover, no one knows.

Hail to Washington, the victor, and to the Bullets who rule the world. And in a town that could use some good news, we now know that we have nothing to fear—not even basketball itself.

A brief note concerning the sport of hockey in Washington, since that is all it usually deserves. Throughout most of the short history of the Washington Capitals hockey team, many have suspected that the players were allergic to frozen water. Also, the confidence of the Capitals' opposing teams was demonstrated by certain psychological ploys used to spook the Capitals' playing. For example, their opponents would do things like having their goalie wear street clothes during the game.

It seemed to me that a team with such an unimaginative name like the Washington Capitals was destined to play in a similar lackluster fashion. When the team was founded, the owner, Abe Pollin, held an area-wide contest to name the team. Out of thousands of entries, he chose the Washington Capitals. Pollin probably named his dog Spot.

Of all the entrepreneurs who ever tried to make a go of it in Washington, the one who infuriated the town the most was a guy named Robert Short. Every time we see weeds growing in the outfield at RFK Stadium, we think of him.

In 1978, just when we had all but forgotten Robert Short, what does he do but announce that he's going to run for the Senate from Minnesota. He never made it; but the story unfolds in this piece which I wrote at the time:

Lately, people have been asking me, in jest, what I think of Richard Nixon's increased public appearances. Do I think he'll run again? Wouldn't it be great to have him back in Washington so we could kick him around once more—silly questions like that. And my answer is that Nixon's return to Washington could be like the triumphant procession from *Aida* compared to the sort of welcome we here would bestow upon Robert Short if he wins the Senate race in Minnesota. Who is Robert Short? He once owned the Washington Senators. Those senators didn't wear three-piece suits, but the uniforms of the major league baseball team of the nation's capital. Mr. Short promised the fans that the team would remain here. After all, Washington, D.C., the citadel of fun and games, should have a big-league team engaged in America's favorite pastime. I'm talking about baseball.

Well, one morning we woke up and discovered that the team was missing. We looked around and saw that Short was gone too. On top of his empty desk we found a note that said, "By the time you read this I'll be in Texas. I've got the team and you'll never get it back." It was signed "Sneaky," which is what we all called him. I admit that such forthright behavior eminently qualifies him for public service, and perhaps he's repented and can show the voters of Minnesota that he is a boy scout. But as of now, he's as welcome in Washington as the locusts. Come to think of it, it's been at least seven years since he left.

There were some fleeting rumors a while back that the colorful baseball maverick Bill Veeck would bring a team to Washington, something we haven't had since the Nixon administration. (Perhaps Mr. Nixon would come back to throw out the first ball, tossing it to his secretary, Rosemary Woods, who would then hide it in her purse.) The legendary Veeck would be great for Washington as a contrast to our oversupply of painfully serious cogs in the government flywheel. Perhaps he would dress the team in short pants, as he almost did in Chicago with the White Sox. I can't imagine the players being too embarrassed—until they come out on the field. Apparently that's what Veeck thought baseball needed—guys weighing 205, wearing handlebar moustaches, chewing tobacco, and dressed in Bermuda shorts.

The phenomenon of the locker room has always left me with the impression that nothing goes on in there that is of benefit to the civilized world. Noisy televised locker-room interviews after the big win always have bad acoustics, the irritating clank of metal on metal, and shouting in the showers. *"Well, ya know, Howard, when we were behind, ya know, three runs in the seventh inning, ya know,—well, it looked, ya know, like we were gonna kiss that pennant, ya know—goodbye!!! Hey, you guys, cut that out!"*

On the same day of the final game of the 1978 World Series, world chess champion Anatoly Karpov retained his title as the final chess match came to an end. Rejoicing in victory, Karpov, still seated at the board, calmly opened a bottle of champagne and poured it over his head.

The highest ideals of sportsmanship and good clean competition always shine at the Olympics. China hates Taiwan, the Soviet Union hates China, everybody hates South Africa, and in 1976 even Canada threw a temper tantrum by objecting to Taiwan's participation in Montreal. It looked as if they would have to establish a demilitarized zone along the 1500-meter track, and if Taiwan was to have any part in the Olympics at all, its athletes would have to sneak over the high hurdles and tiptoe over the finish line. Canada's proposal to the Taiwanese was preposterous: "Okay, you can play, but if anybody asks, you are Puerto Ricans."

The 1976 conventions were going on at the time, and President Jerry Ford, fighting for the nomination, took the time to come to Taiwan's defense, having been told that the team contained two uncommitted delegates. This was the second time the United States applied sportsmanship in its treatment of Taiwan. The first time occurred several years earlier when we shot-putted them out of the United Nations.

When the Winter Olympics of 1980 were held, darned if the same thing didn't happen. By then, the ceremonial cross-country dumping of Taiwan had become a regularly scheduled event. As part of the opening festivities at Lake Placid, New York, the American officials in their gaily-colored costumes artfully snatched the flagpole bearing the flag of Taiwan and hurled it for a record 35 feet into a snowbank. This was followed by the equally thrilling Egg-on-the-Face Classic. The officials, having perfected their timing since their last performance in '76, bravely challenged the Taiwan team to surrender its pride. But, the stubborn Taiwanese refused as always. The officials then employed the next exercise. This was the very tricky extending of the Pathetic Compromise. The Pathetic Compromise was the challenge to the members of the Taiwan team to give up their nationality for two weeks and become honorary citizens of the village of Lake Placid. As Lake Placidians, the ex-Taiwanese athletes would have been entitled to a free oil change at Ernie's Texaco—as well as a hot chocolate on the house at the Adirondack Diner.

In 1980, however, the dumping of Taiwan had a new twist. The officials rescued the Taiwan flag from the snowbank and, running it across the field, presented it to the team of the People's Republic of China as a reward for their boycotting of the games for 30 years.

Of course, we pulled out of the Summer Olympics in Moscow because the Russians invaded Afghanistan searching for a warm water port—preferably New Orleans. NBC, originally scheduled to broadcast the Games, wasn't hurt too badly because they had a no-risk insurance policy with Lloyd's of Cleveland. This company is for those who have been turned down by Mutual of Tijuana.

Believe it or not, there are still a few of us left in these United States in 1980 who have no desire to engage in anything remotely connected with running, jogging, sprinting, or conveying oneself on foot in any manner save that of the leisurely ambling stroll. To say that the jogger is a menace to society would be excessively kind, as they block streets and sidewalks, huffing and loping and smelling up the landscape with their sweat-soaked socks and warm-up suits.

Are joggers taxed? No. Why not have license plates on them? Do they use gasoline which helps the gross national product? No. All they do is support the sneaker industry, a good portion of which is Korean. Need I say more? Do they make us feel guilty? Yes. But not me, not any more. I don't even feel conscience-stricken about my increasing temptation to chase joggers with my car and watch the broken field running as I bear down on them. Now that's recreation! That's sport! You should be here in Washington at noon and drive by the Pentagon. Why, these joggers run up over your hood when they should be inside planning wars.

A favorite athletic endeavor among officeholders is the fine old sport of fishing. If they are not engaged in the figurative meaning of fishing ("that committee is merely conducting a fishing expedition") then they actually do head for the peace and solace of a line and sinker by a peaceful stream.

Eisenhower had his golf; Kennedy had his sailing; Johnson had his horses; Nixon had his tape recorder; and Carter's fishing captured the nation's imagination when he did it from a canoe. Now right away we have a problem. Does anyone really fish from a canoe? Aren't you supposed to sit quietly in a canoe and make as few motions as possible? Pretty risky for a president. Any historian will tell you about the time President William Henry Harrison was fishing in a canoe with his vice president, John Tyler. The darned thing tipped over. Hence the expression "Tippecanoe and Tyler, too."

But I digress. As the story about Carter went on, all of a sudden an angry rabbit started to swim toward the president's canoe, perhaps fleeing from a predator (do they mean a Republican?). The rabbit was said to be making a hissing sound. My friends, we now have an administration that asks us to believe that you can fish from a canoe and that rabbits can swim and hiss. Are we also to believe that snakes can hop?

As the rabbit approached, the president began striking at it with a paddle. (You thought he was without one, didn't you?) The result of this incident was that the National Paddle Association came to the defense with a slogan that said, "Paddles don't kill rabbits, people kill rabbits."

I suppose I should conclude this salute to sport by saying something good about at least one athletic endeavor. (This tendency toward fairness is imbedded in me after years of receiving letters saying, "Why don't you say something *good* about America?" It's a feeling that comes over me from time to time but, like a minor headache, passes.) This is going to require as much courage as admitting to not owning sneakers, since the sport I am fond of is looked upon disparagingly in certain circles. Here goes. I, uh, like to bowl. Now wait a minute . . . Before you conjure up prejudices of unlettered, beer-belching brawlers on a Saturday night in a northeastern neighborhood ten-pin tap room, let me say that there is a poetic, even spiritual side to bowling.

Each of the defiant pins represents a painful aspect of life—poverty, ignorance, greed, hypocrisy, your boss, and so on. They dare you to strike them down. The smooth, perfect spheroid cradled in your hands is like the cannonballs fired at Appomattox and York town to still the enemy and to right the wrongs of an unsettled world. Released, the ball follows its course straight and true. At the moment of impact, if all goes well, the joyous clank of toppling pins signals the victory and triumph surely felt by Douglas Mac-Arthur as he waded ashore in the Philippines. One can almost hear the trumpeted heraldry of the "Charge of the Light Brigade" when one scores high in bowling. Of course, there are times when you throw nothing but gutter balls, and then all you can hear is the juke box playing "D-I-V-O-R-C-E" by Tammy Wynette.

Jimmy Carter taught me to bowl. All those speeches of his about how Washington was out of touch with the real Americans drove me in pursuit of a sport other than those associated with politicians—golf and tennis. Bowling in Washington is just as popular as everywhere else, but the city nevertheless is perceived by the rest of the country as consisting of either high-crime ghettos or Georgetown salons, with foppish carousers attending an endless round of cocktail parties where the hors d'oeurves are made of ultrasuede and the dogs wear Gucci flea collars.

This image of the nation's capital is why Washington-based newspaper columnists believe they get a truer picture of Middle America if they write a column on the mood of the nation from Iowa. All they have to do is visit a bowling alley just a few miles from their office.

So in defense of bowling, let me say that there is an erroneous perception of the image of the bowler. Golfers and tennis players, those snob sports, cast disparaging glances at we who love bowling. Too many of those elitists are of the patently false opinion that the bowler is unsophisticated, unpolished, and crude. Well, I'm a bowler, and I say that's bullshit.

8. What Do the Lone Ranger, Superman, Radio City Music Hall, and Bert Parks Have in Common?

There comes a time in the course of human events when the public turns away from alarming headlines, the thought of bread lines, receding hairlines, and other depressions and rallies in support of certain individuals or institutions that have been badly treated. This is called feeling better by helping others. In the past several years, four landmarks of our cultural landscape have been threatened with either extinction or neglect, only to be saved in an eleventh-hour rescue mission by the public. The basic good in all of us can sense that an institution is worth saving. Such was the case when we, as a people, raised our voices and saved the wrecker's ball from toppling the Lone Ranger, Superman, Radio City Music Hall, and Bert Parks.

Superman must have known how Al Jolson felt when, back in the late forties, the movie *The Jolson Story* came out and introduced the singer to a whole new generation at a time when he was nearly forgotten. There was a tremendous revival in Jolson's career. The same kind of thing happened a few years ago to Superman.

Superman was getting old and he knew it. It had come to the point where he was chasing only small-time crooks and the buildings he was leaping over were more medium-sized than tall; and even with those, it took more than just a single bound. It also had been years since he ran faster than a speeding bullet; in fact, if he beat the Amtrak to New Haven it was considered a good day. In the desperation that comes to many of us, he looked in the mirror one day and said, "Nobody cares about fighting for truth, justice, and the American way any more. It's this damn 'Me' decade."

Apparently, someone out in Hollywood got to thinking that there was a whole new generation out there that just might take to a good, clean, honest American superhero for a change. "Maybe these ill-mannered, dope-smoking, mop-haired rock-star punks have run their course," he thought, "and the time is right to retell the Superman story in a new movie, using the latest in special effects and stereophonic sound."

Well, tell that story they did. The picture was a smash, not only with the kids, but also with other folks, because it had a degree of sophistication that surpassed any television series or comic books of bygone days. As for Superman himself, he soon moved out of his sad little third-floor walk-up into new digs out on the Coast. The wrinkles in his face seemed to disappear, and he was leaping those tall buildings with the old single bound again. In fact, it wasn't taking him nearly as long to perform those other physical feats either, if you know what I mean.

The movie itself, made by Warner Brothers, starts the story at Superman's birthplace, the planet Krypton. His father, Marlon Brando, the former Don of a Mafia family, has moved there earlier to escape the Feds. He has this cute little baby who he thinks would be better off living in Kansas. The kid comes hurling from this other planet and plops right into the middle of Kansas, which is like watching *The Wizard of Oz* run backward. This kid proves to be different, not because he can kick a football five miles or lift up a truck with one hand—no, he's different because, although there is literally nothing he can't do, he chooses to live in Kansas. When he grows up, however, he moves to the big city and becomes a meek, mild-mannered reporter. A meek reporter? This movie really is a fantasy. When Superman has difficulty in dealing with some of life's problems on Earth, he seeks advice from Brando, who is now living in New Orleans, where we see him wearing a torn undershirt and drinking beer, having changed his name to Stanley Kowalski.

We see all the familiar tricks in the movie. Superman stops bullets with his chest, catches a crashing helicopter with one hand, and in a brand new gimmick pulls the San Andreas fault together, which eventually leads to his defeating Jerry Brown for governor of California. Conceding victory, Brown bitterly tells reporters, "I never thought the public would fall for such demagoguery."

At last report, they were planning a sequel in which Superman would perform his most amazing feat. With one hand, he would raise the stock of his producers, Warner Communications, to one thousand dollars a share.

Of all the *causes célèbres* we have seen over the years, none is more heart-rending than the case of the actor Clayton Moore. After Moore had played the Lone Ranger for thirty years, a younger actor went to court to claim the title of Lone Ranger for himself. The judge, ruling in favor of the younger man, ordered Moore to stop wearing his mask. This was the kind of situation that triggers the public's imagination into sympathizing with an older, more venerable institution, in this case, Clayton Moore, the "real" Lone Ranger.

John Wayne had just passed away; we had a president widely perceived to be weak; and it seemed that then, more than ever before, we needed a steady, mature, 64-old-year-old Lone Ranger. Feeling badly about the whole situation, I wrote the following on Clayton Moore's behalf:

"Is there no room in this disco-crazed, throw-away society for any vestiges of stability and tradition? By demasking the Lone Ranger you demask the goddess of justice and you deny an American institution his inalienable right to life, liberty, and the pursuit of outlaws. As you cannot have two popes, you cannot have two Lone Rangers. You can only have one Lone Ranger. If you have more than one ranger, those rangers, being plural, cannot be 'lone,' can they? So let's support the Lone Ranger, our smallest minority group. And if you can read this and listen to the "William Tell Overture" at the same time without choking up, you have a heart of stone."

As the hands of the clock slowly crept toward midnight, a silent crowd stood outside the governor's mansion in Albany, New York, waiting for the decision. In Times Square, to the south, another equally silent gathering stared up at the electronic news flash sign for word on the fate of Radio City Music Hall. Finally, word came of the governor's reprieve, saving the Music Hall and the Rockettes, if only temporarily.

For more than 40 years, the Radio City Music Hall has stood as a palace of good, clean family entertainment. The Music Hall always had a long line outside waiting to see the latest hit movie and dazzling stage show complete with that chorus of apple-cheeked, all-American dancers, the Rockettes.

But the realities of New York's financial situation, along with the changing face of Manhattan in general, brought hard times to the Music Hall and it was facing having to be closed. There was a lot of haranguing about why can't a nice place like this thrive and what has happened to our values? It became evident that the very proper old hall had no right being amid the results of urban deterioration. Benefits were held and editorials were written, and through the machinery of influence and various loopholes, it was allowed to carry on and is still thriving; at least, as of this writing.

You might say that the Rockettes had been guilty of being offensively wholesome. Their behavior on stage was outdated and not in step with today's popularity for X-rated attractions. Surely there must have been complaints from the Times Square entrepreneurs about the Music Hall's insufficient trash, public cleanliness, blatant lack of filth, and numerous violations of the Times Square Code of Sleaze.

"Your Honor," the public prosecutor might have said, "this type of entertainment may go over in Dubuque, but this is sophisticated New York." Referring specifically to the Music Hall's Easter Pageant, the prosecutor might have continued, "In order to meet the standards of popular entertainment in today's world, those Easter bunnies are going to have to do something sexier than just hippity-hoppiting around on the stage."

Barely minutes before the Rockettes were to dance their last mile, they heard from the governor. They would be given one more year while New York City decided on the alternatives to a death sentence. One compromise suggested was that the Music Hall could feature a clean show and an X-rated movie, or a dirty show and a G-rated movie. But as for a clean show with a G-rated movie, they'd have to move the whole six thousand seats out of town. Probably all the way to Dubuque.

"There she is, Miss America. There she is, our *ideeel* ..."

Ah, who could ever forget that song, sung by one man, and one man alone, Bert Parks. That Pepsodent smile, the jet-black Corfam hair, the voice as wrinkled as his face. What a job he had! One night a year, directing traffic on the stage in Atlantic City, the site of the Miss America Pageant.

When it was announced that because Bert Parks was 65 years old, they weren't renewing his contract, Americans momentarily forgot about Iran, Afghanistan, and 18 percent inflation, and cried out, "Bert Parks fired? They might as well strip-mine Mount Rushmore." Our nation became united in its indignation for the first time since the firing of the Lone Ranger, and we took to the streets. As church bells rang for Bert every hour on the hour, everyone was sadly aware that this was just one more example of the constant chipping away at the foundations of the republic. I suppose we should have known that once they took the prayers out of the schools, it would be only a matter of time before Bert Parks would be forced to stop singing the one song he had ever learned.

As I said, there are certain times when the people of this nation will rise up and say no to that which they are told is inevitable, and this was one of those times. The mood was best described by a bumper sticker of the time: "Save the redwoods, save the whales, save Bert Parks."

But Bert stayed fired. And they hired Ron Ely, who had played Tarzan on TV, to be the host. I guess we can look forward to seeing him dressed in a loincloth, swinging from a vine, as he sings "Here she comes, Miss America." Of course, we know who'll win the contest—who else would Tarzan pick but some beauty named Jane?

9. Read This Chapter and Call Me in the Morning

You can call me Ray.   —GAMMA

I wanted to write a chapter on doctors and another one on golf, when I realized I could handle both themes by writing a chapter only on doctors. This is a sneaky way of offering the opinion that golfing and doctoring go together, usually on Wednesday afternoons. But we won't belabor the point, as the indictment of the Sneads of the scalpel has been overdone.

A surprising announcement came out of a meeting of surgeons several years ago that, contrary to popular opinion, playing golf was not as beneficial to the heart as the more strenuous sports, such as squash. (That makes sense when you consider that you have never heard of any squash widows.) This announcement did not suggest that doctors would be quitting golf in droves, however difficult playing in a drove might be.

That there is only minimal beneficial effect of golf on the heart must be unsettling information to the poor duffer who thought he was forever keeping the grim reaper off the Fairway of Life by playing. No longer can these guys say in good conscience, "Sure, I shot in the high nineties, but take a look at this EKG." Actually, a bad golfer does his heart more good than a superior golfer. Those long hunt-and-find walks in the woods can be very invigorating.

Being of rather sound mind and body, it has been my good luck to come into contact with doctors for the most part on a professional basis. I occasionally speak to their groups and lobbying organizations around the country. (Once out of their white jackets, doctors resemble a roomful of congressmen.) Which is why I find the television show "M*A*S*H" unbelievable, although highly entertaining; I never met anyone like Hawkeye or B.J. Hunnicut at the Legislative Conference of the American Medical Political Action Committee (AMPAC).

The doctor can use his title as a shield against the charges leveled at him over the years. Medicine is absolutely the most authoritative of all the professions. The overriding fact is that the doctor will always have his specialty and will know what we don't know. Therefore, the doctor will always be superior—and will often act that way. With the politician, the lawyer, or even your plumber or bookmaker, you can sometimes fake it by showing off a little knowledge, but with the doctor, never.

No wonder getting that title means so much. A Ph.D who doesn't know asparagus about medicine seldom corrects anyone who thinks he's an M.D. In some areas, even the local druggist calls himself "doctor." "The doctor will see you now" is always whispered by his white-clad receptionist with great reverence, as if ushering you into the presence of some living god.

Other keepers of this perpetual flame of respect are the front line troops of the American Medical Association—the aforementioned AMPAC. They are the Green Berets of medicine, running skirmishes through the halls of Congress, successfully spearheading the attack on The Enemy—national health insurance.

The supply line of food and ammunition (money) to virtually every member of Congress is in keeping with the old adage of warfare that an army travels on its stomach. As a derelict knows that he can always get a bowl of soup at the Gospel Mission, any congressman, Democrat or Republican, can always count on a campaign donation from AMPAC. No one is refused. The first thing a freshman congressman learns on the day he arrives at his new job is that an apple a day won't keep AMPAC away. This, of course, is legitimate lobbying procedure on behalf of the medical profession, and I like to think of it as First Aid.

Premed students should give serious thought to specializing in political action. Sure, surgery and podiatry are lucrative, but a career in lobbying can be very rewarding. You get to travel and meet famous politicians, and you don't have to get depressed being around a lot of sick people. If you wish to go into medicine, but faint at the sight of blood, I suggest becoming a lobbyist—or an osteopath. Of course, there's nothing to say that the AMPAC doctor can't occasionally drop by his office and see a patient or two just to keep in practice, so to speak.

There is another type of physician who is uncomfortable around hospitals, and that type is the Doctor of Broadcasting (M.D.B.) His instruments are the TV camera and the microphone, and during his operations, the only sponge used is for the application of pancake make-up.

You've seen them on the tube: "Ask the Doctor," "Doctor's Housecall," and so on. They're articulate, as handsome as anchormen, and can make you forget wars and taxes by reminding you of your gallstones.

Some news rooms also have a resident psychologist in attendance but these are especially found on local radio talk shows. We had such a show in Washington, called "Psychological Grab Bag," and I think its competitor on a rival station was called "Depression Merry-Go-Round." On the opening show of the "Grab Bag," a man called in seeking help for alcoholism. The host-shrink drew on her expertise and said, "Mister, you should stop drinking." (And if you can't, let's have a drink together and talk about why you can't stop.)

The argument can be made that offering free medical advice on the air is a helpful service, especially to those who cannot afford today's rising health costs. Such an argument is valid, but only up to a point. The TV doctor will provide only half a service until we also have the TV druggist. Since a trip to the doctor is always accompanied by a trip to a druggist, the same should apply to television.

Here's how it would work: On the "Today Show," Tom Brokaw introduces Dr. Art Uline and his partner, Irving Rexall, the famed proprietor of Irving's Pharmacy located on the ground floor of the RCA Building. Art Uline kicks it off: "Heart attacks can be bothersome but also can be avoided by regular exercise, stopping smoking, staying on a low-cholesterol diet, and of course, daily dosages of that very helpful drug, digitalis. My advice is free, and so is the digitalis at Irving's Pharmacy, right, Irving?"

"That's right, Art. Simply drop by my store, mention that Art Uline sent you, and you'll receive a bottle of digitalis on the house."

It's not really on the house, because, as part of the plan, Irving is reimbursed by NBC in the same manner they pay Art Uline for his services.

The role of the drug manufacturers may not be what most of us imagine. Very few people outside the profession have ever had the occasion to thumb through the in-house magazines read by doctors, or have seen the exhibits at a medical convention. These give you the instant impression that though it's the doctor who tells you what's wrong with you, it's the pharmaceutical companies who tell the doctor how to cure it.

"Name a disease, and we've got something for it," hawk their ads. "Seen any goiters lately? Stock up on Zebutrex® now!"

"You never know when a patient will walk in looking like this" (we see a picture of a man whose face is contorted in obvious pain). "Recognize it? Is that chronic hypertension or is that chronic hypertension? Take advantage of our year-end closeout special on Spantalebutons® now!

"And remember, for every ten prescriptions for Spantalebutons®, you get 100 Valiums FREE!"

In one year, drug manufacturers give out an average of 1,159,-278,328 free samples of their prescription products to doctors. I suppose that's why doctors don't make house calls anymore. It sounds to me like they're too stoned to drive. It's amazing that a doctor can lean against the door of a closet in his office jam-packed with free drugs and complain about socialized medicine.

When a doctor attends a convention, he is constantly invited to such gala affairs as the Valium Happy Hour and Luau and the Benedril Bingo Party. Invitations await his arrival to "attend tonight's Madcap Darvon and Coricidin Charleston Contest."

My doctor was so grateful for the free samples that he overdid his gratitude to the manufacturer. He once wrote a prescription that said, "Take 12 a day, forever, and order extras for your friends."

Several years ago, a doctor working for the government threw the profession into a dither when he took much less than a hard line against smoking. In fact, this doctor—whose name was, and I suppose still is, Gori—decided that some cigarettes were tolerable. Well, you should have heard the cheering at the Tobacco Is Wonderful Institute. But all was gloom over at Chuck That Butt Inc., where Joe Califano, proprietor, sentenced Dr. Gori to four tours in a small elevator with three cigar smokers puffing at full throttle.

Dr. Gori listed twenty-seven brands that have a tolerable level ranging from twenty-three a day down to a three-a-day danger point. Refraining from citing actual brand names, we will use fictitious ones for reasons of propriety and fear of lawsuits. According to Dr. Gori, if you puff away on eighteen Laughing Lung Menthols a day, fine, but number 19 could mean trouble. Smoke Popsickle Puff 100s and you can have twenty-three a day, but watch out for Soot Lites, warns the doctor, because three a day means a quick farewell, and no ifs, ands, or butts about it.

Enough about the dangers of smoking. Let's talk about a paradise where even the thought of sickness and disease doesn't exist. It is a carefree place where never a discouraging word about cigarettes is heard. This place is the Tobacco Is Wonderful Institute, where the motto is, "There is nothing wrong with cigarettes—it's the matches that getcha." A terrible slogan, to be sure. I suggested a somewhat more realistic approach—"Cigarettes are as American as emphysema and apple pie"—but they were coughing so loudly they couldn't hear me.

Another medical proclamation I believe we all could have done without came from a number of prominent hospitals, announcing a technique enabling doctors to determine the sex of a baby before it is born, so that the mother, wanting a boy instead of a girl, could opt for aborting the fetus of the unwanted sex.

In defense of this practice, the doctors say that the mothers in these cases might have an abortion anyway, but if they knew whether it was a boy or a girl, they might not. Some might call this an expansion of the right to choose. I call it fetus roulette. But at least it will take away some of the surprise the expectant father must endure in the waiting room. Now the doctor enters and announces, "Congratulations—it's a boy. But, of course, you knew that." It's really a pity that hospitals can't use the sales pitch of the fast-food chain to proclaim, "Have it your way at Riverside General."

If you don't think you're having it your way, you can call your physician and get a recorded announcement: "The doctor is on the line with God at the moment—please leave your name and number."

In opposition to the views of a number of doctors and judges, the Supreme Court ruled last year that laetrile, derived from apricot pits, was an illegal drug. The reason given by the Court was that nobody had been able to prove that it wasn't harmful.

The decision opens the possibility of Federal agents breaking into someone's house and staging a laetrile bust. Imagine two narcs frisking a suspect: "Nothing here but pot, hash, and cocaine, Charlie. He's clean." Marijuana is acceptable because they can't prove that it's harmful. And laetrile is now illegal because they can't prove that it *isn't* harmful. Of course, cigarettes are legal because the tobacco lobby is more powerful than the apricot pit lobby.

Meanwhile, as the debate over federal health care continues, many people obstinately continue to get sick without having enough money to pay for it. For these thoughtless people who refuse to be healthy, there could be an alternate plan—no-frills surgery.

There's no reason why hospitals can't offer the American public what it wants at a price it can afford. No-frills surgery provides low prices with luxury options available at extra cost. Let's take it by category: for an appendectomy, for example, with no-frills anesthesia, you get your choice of a silver bullet, whiskey, or a block of wood to bite down on. For abdominal surgery, you may select a scalpel or a cuticle remover. For a broken arm you may choose to set your bone in fiberglass, a plaster cast, or a splint made from a bandana and coat hanger.

There are also many more ways to cut the costs of a hospital visit. For example, in the no-frills recuperating rooms, you make your own bed and go home on the day of the operation—or stay at the Y. Bandages are an option, and if you don't want them, your wounds can be bound with paper and twine. Since hospital gowns and linen are costly, all operations will be performed strictly "come as you are." Because, remember, "as you are" is why you're there.

When I first heard about the imaginative course at the University of Iowa's College of Dentistry called "Children and Dental Fear," I thought: At last, a course for dentists to overcome their fear of children. For years, it has been assumed that it was the child's fear of the dentist that made the profession so difficult. Dentists tried everything. Some dentists decorated their offices to resemble circus midways, with calliope music, balloons, trained seals, and juggling hygienists. The dentists would wear clown suits and make their drills look like cowboy guns to amuse the little tykes and take away their fear.

But recently, dentists have begun admitting that it is their fear of children that drives them to the golf course when they should be working. What are they afraid of? Well, when you think about it, there are a number of reasons to fear children—sixteen on the bottom and sixteen on the top. Yes, those little nippers can bite.

So, if you are the wife or mother of a dentist, you can help him by never speaking in a negative way about children, even though treating them these days is like pulling teeth.

Lest it appear that I am down on all doctors, there are two specialists for whom I have complete sympathy. They are pediatricians and psychiatrists.

To begin with, the pediatrician would surely be a much happier person if he never had to talk to an adult. A particular problem is what is called in the trade a "PJM"—the Pediatrician Junkie Mother, who, when the temperature first dips into the sixties, calls the doctor in a panic and asks, "Should little Seymour wear a hat to school?" Then there are the mothers who never know when the child should be weaned, as it were, away from the baby doctor. Often the youngster is brought into the office by his mother, and the doctor says, "Okay, cowboy, jump up on the table and let's have a look at you," when the "cowboy" is nineteen and probably taller than the pediatrician.

However, one of the baby doctor's biggest problems has to do with how he spends his off-duty hours. Remember, he is in a kindergarten atmosphere all day long. Portraits of Popeye and Wimpy adorn the walls of his office. The chairs are hobby horses. The reading matter in his waiting room offers a wide selection from *The Little Engine That Could* to *Raggedy Andy and the*

AND THAT REMINDS ME...

The Senate has voted to put "Hazardous to Your Health" labels on bottles of booze. Well, that solves the alcoholism problem—now on to global unrest.

The U.S. Senate has voted to place a label on liquor bottles saying: "Warning! The consumption of alcoholic beverages can be hazardous to your health." Well, since this will do about as much good as the labels on cigarettes, I suggest forming the Bureau of Hazard Warning Label Specifications of the Department of HEW. There is an urgent need for such labels on many items such as sneakers which say: "Warning! Sneakers are not to be jogged in while in the path of an oncoming truck!" How about rock albums having a label on them? "Warning! Playing this record at high volume can turn your parents into irrational monsters." And perhaps newborn babies could have a label stuck on them which says: "Warning! Caring for babies can rob you of the social life you had before you stupidly got married when you were too young." And, in springtime, lawn fertilizer could have a label which says: "Warning! Trying to have a greener lawn than the guy across the street can give you ulcers, as opposed to surrendering to the dandelions and weeds." I picture a warning on men's hair formula: "Warning! Getting rid of the gray can bring on delusions that all the young girls in the office think you look like Burt Reynolds, while in fact you're starting to resemble Sydney Greenstreet."

Talking Turtle. Little wonder that at an all-adult evening gathering, a pediatrician might greet someone with "Golly, gee, how are we today?" and then stroll over to the bar and order a Shirley Temple.

There's a unique problem of psychiatrists that is seldom noticed. Even though they are at present knocking down at least $60 per 45-minute session, their tax situation in regard to office equipment is unfavorable. Other doctors have many machines and instruments that are tax-deductible tools of the trade. The psychiatrist has only the couch and the Kleenex. There are notebooks, of course, but I have begun to have suspicions about what notations are actually made in them.

During the Watergate period, when the office of Daniel Ells-
berg's psychiatrist was broken into, I asked a psychiatrist friend of
mine about how much material an analyst could accumulate on
any given patient over several years. The doctor thought it over for
a moment and said, "Well, sometimes it could be up to a page and
a half."

In the late seventies, *Time* magazine reported in a cover article
that psychiatry itself was going through a depression, suggesting
that this was due to people opting for trendy shrink-your-own-
head therapies instead of the more orthodox treatments. You can
imagine how difficult it must be for a high-priced analyst trying to
compete with an ad that says: "Hey, there, sickie! Now you can
kick that annoying homicidal manic tendency on your lunch
break!"

Pop therapy is all around us. Perhaps establishment psychiatry's
days became numbered when somebody invented the Smile but-
ton. How can the disciples of Sigmund Freud compete with the
phenomenon of do-it-yourself mood altering at home. How can
their fees stand up against the price of self-help books with titles
like *I'm into Me 'Cause That's Where I'm At* or *In Touch with
Myself While Searching Within* or *Running in Place Alone?*

So pity the poor psychiatrist. He went to school all those years,
studied hard, entered an honorable profession, joined the country
club, and now he may have to close up shop because a good old-
fashioned depression is becoming harder to come by. And do you
know why? Because too many of us believe we can really "have a
nice day" if we read the right book or learn how to work our
mood-changing rings so that we are never blue.

10. Instant Impressions (Just Add Water)

Now for some rapid fire, top of my head, instant reflections on a few people—in and out of Washington. Some of them are friends; some are mere acquaintances. Some I have met, and some I have not. Some might have met me but probably won't admit it.

SENATOR EDWARD KENNEDY: He and I are exactly the same age—and if I were president, wouldn't that scare the hell out of you?

RONALD REAGAN: Think back to the first time you ever saw him—in the picture frame department at Woolworth's, right? His picture was always between Gale Storm and Walter Pidgeon.

WALTER MONDALE: When I started saying that in California they thought Mondale was a little town outside Pasadena, he said he liked the line and wanted more like it. So I said that he once attended a Mondale family reunion in Minnesota and that he needed a name tag. He also liked that one. Then I said that Mondale was spelled M-U-N-D-A-N-E. He didn't like that one.

JIMMY CARTER: His first crisis occurred at a press conference when a reporter said that he had a question about Rhodesia. Carter said, "At last a question about something other than Bert Lance. What's your question?" The reporter said, "Does Bert Lance have a bank in Rhodesia?"

WILLIAM F. BUCKLEY: Probably the only person in the world who would work in a word like "solipsistic"—while calling his dog.

SENATOR EDMUND MUSKIE: When he ran for president, his friends called him Lincoln without the stove-pipe hat. His enemies called him the stove-pipe hat without Lincoln.

GERALD FORD: His clumsiness was always exaggerated. Although, one time, during the Bicentennial, he was officiating at a ceremony in the National Archives Building honoring the Constitution and he tripped over the Preamble.

CONGRESSMAN MORRIS UDALL: The wittiest man in Congress. Wouldn't it be funny if we found out that his gag writer was his insurance salesman?

SENATOR S. I. HAYAKAWA: The tap dancing mascot of the Senate. Tourists go to the Capitol Building just to watch him sleep. He may wake up long enough to do a remake of the Gene Kelly movie, *Singing in the Rain,* in Japan.

HAMILTON JORDAN: That cocaine charge was unfair, and Jordan was justifiably angry. "That's a lie," he snorted.

HENRY KISSINGER: At a Gridiron Dinner with Kissinger, Rosalynn Carter said to him—"You Yankees sure talk funny."

SENATOR DANIEL PATRICK MOYNIHAN: One of my favorite senators. He is very intelligent and tough, but for some reason he looks like he wears pajamas with the feet in them.

RICHARD NIXON: His resignation made me very sad. I had to go back to writing my own material.

MADALYN MURRAY O'HARE: Atheists the world over should be proud to have her as their Mother Superior.

MARTIN AGRONSKY: The veteran newsman opens his weekly talk show by listing all of the troubles of the world, looking as if he holds himself personally responsible.

DAVID ROCKEFELLER: I always thought any one of the Rockefellers would make a good president. After all, anyone who owns something should be permitted to run it.

ALEXANDER SOLZHENITSYN: He once told the graduating class at Harvard, "You Americans are getting fat and lazy." He got no applause on that line. The students were asleep.

ELIZABETH TAYLOR: Her life as the wife of a senator must be some kind of dream. The way I see it, a few years ago she was half-dozing on a yacht with an assortment of beautiful people. In a flash, she woke up and found herself standing in the reception line at a political fund raiser in Falls Church, Virginia, holding a Ritz cracker smeared with Velveeta. She must have wondered what she was doing there. The appearance of happiness amid such surroundings means she is an even better actress than we thought she was.

GEORGE WILL: The very able and respected columnist articulates traditional conservative doctrine most succinctly. The son Ronald Reagan never had.

ANDREW YOUNG: His leaving the U.N. caused a serious rift between blacks and Jews in America. At one point it got so bad Sammy Davis, Jr. wouldn't eat with himself.

MSTISLAV ROSTROPOVICH: I sometimes wonder if we realize how lucky we are to have him as the conductor of the National Symphony. Few talents in this town are so instantly discernible. The moment he begins to play the cello, you know you are hearing the best in the field—as opposed to hearing a speech by Senator "Scoop" Jackson.

JACK ANDERSON: I never met a Syndicated Mormon Muckraker I didn't like. Although sometimes the old rake comes up muckless.

SARAH MCLENDON: Watching a White House press conference without an outrageous question hollered out by Screamin' Sarah is like watching a batter being purposely walked by the pitcher. The man is getting off too easy.

ALICE ROOSEVELT LONGWORTH: I never met her but I had always wanted to. Seventy years after her father, Theodore Roosevelt left office, she was still in Washington holding court. One of her wickedly impish sayings was embroidered on a legendary needlepoint pillow of hers—"If you can't say something good about anybody, have a seat right here by me." Who knows? Perhaps a mid-Twenty-first Century Amy Carter will be issuing periodical scourges upon the survivors of the Kennedy Clan.

11. Sexual Politics, Domestic Affairs, and Federal Frigidity

Power is the ultimate aphrodisiac. —HENRY KISSINGER

Where are the broads? —H. JORDAN

Sex as discussed in this chapter will only be in a political context. That's the only way in which the subject is presented in Washington. I'll arouse no prurient interest here, no lurid prose; I'm incapable of it. I try, but invariably I shift back to dreary, unsexy Washington: "The filmy silkiness of her blouse stretched taut against her heaving breasts as, with lips half-parted, she whispered, 'Did you see what Evans and Novak said this morning?' And when it was over and they both lay still, smoking a cigarette, he leaned over and tenderly announced that as soon as he got to the office he would draw up another amendment to his federal water pollution control bill."

There never seems to be any free discussion of pure sex in Washington (or impure sex, either) other than how it might relate to the government. Any conversation centered around a highly passionate novel or motion picture is always contained within a larger conversation about, say, some Supreme Court ruling on the subject. Adultery? Fornication? Group sex? In Washington, we don't pay much attention to such things until they are connected with our newsmakers. In fact, a congressman wallowing in immorality would not gain our attention unless he turned out to be an important committee chairman. A voluptuous secretary typing 12 words a minute being paid 25 thou a year? Not sexy. What is sexy is that her boss, Congressman Wayne Hays, was a real power in Congress and all the Capitol voyeurs were titilated by spying on *him*, not her, in the boudoir.

The members of Congress getting themselves tangled in such iniquities have grown fewer in number, but there was a case a few years ago when someone discovered that according to the Constitution, a congressman could be arrested only for treason or felonies. So when one was arrested for soliciting a prostitute, his lawyer could have demanded that under the Constitution, proof be established that the congressman forced the prostitute to overthrow the government. Such proof could be interpreted as meaning that the "customer" had to do the suggesting, such as rolling down the car window and saying "Hey, sweetheart, here's twenty bucks for a little treason." It also follows that he could, under the Constitution, be arrested for suggesting unnatural acts such as sedition. Let it be said that, like everyone else, our lawmakers are only human and sometimes will give in to temptations of the flesh and wander from the straight and narrow. When this occurs, they needn't worry, so long as they have had their congressional immunity shots—and loyalty oaths.

On occasion, the federal government and sex are coupled with interesting results. Such was the case when at one time, the Justice Department became the proud owner of a rather sleazy topless bar in a somewhat neglected section of downtown Washington. It seems there was this guy who stood convicted of embezzling money from the government office where he worked. He had purchased with some of these funds a place called the Lone Star Beef House. The name wasn't exactly fitting, since the main attraction of the establishment was not the cuisine, but the half-clad and completely un-clad exotic dancers who began performing every weekday at noon.

One of the items the Justice Department received as partial compensation was the bar. The government ran the place for 18 months before it was auctioned off at, uncharacteristically, a substantial profit. So you see, we *can* balance the budget and even show a surplus if we use a little fiscal responsibility, like that demonstrated at the Lone Beef House Institute of Economics.

The idea of the government running a topless bar conjures up a vision of what it must have been like to administer it as a part of the bureaucracy. Imagine a memo written to the manager in typical federalese gobbledegook:

MEMO

Pursuant to House, Beef (Lone Star) 14–106 Guidelines and Dynamics for Position Evaluation—Orchestration of Ecdysiast Interpretations Therein Thereof:

The performance standards shall be determined on a daily basis by the Justice Department designated Lone Star Beef House Administrator, General Services Administration. The prevailing thematic austerity configuration within the G.S.A. and its environs dictates that the necessity exists for the avoidance of Nixon administration iniquities and therefore the rules and regulations of the aforementioned Lone Star Beef House would be to negate at all costs any hint of a cover-up.

The Lone Star Beef House still flourishes, and on your next trip to the nation's capital you might wish to go there, not to ogle the girls but rather to view the clientele. Many of them are respectable-looking, upright, serious citizens. Leave your camera at the hotel, though, because the sight of one causes these gentlemen to head for the door. You see, the Lone Star Beef House is just a few doors down from the FBI.

The Bureau always has seemed to have more than a passing interest in sex. Consider, for example, that on an apparently slow day, agents raided a massage parlor just outside of town. This episode wasn't exactly in the great tradition gunning down John Dillinger in front of the Biograph Theatre in Chicago, but rather the slapping of a citation of Trixie Latour in front of the Midnight Love Nest in Alexandria, Virginia. (The names have been changed to protect the lecherous.)

Reading about the raid, I assumed there would be a resulting set of federal guidelines on the parlors. For example, all words of enticement would have to be deleted from the names of massage parlors such as "ecstacy" and "foxy." No more Cupid's Delight or Suzie's House of Fantasy. From now on, less sensuous titles would be used, such as Edna's Gymnasium, or Matilda's Reading Room, The Dank Museum, or perhaps Fred's Stockade. Under the FBI ruling, the customer would be led into a brightly-lit room where the temperature was 47 degrees. As an FBI-suggested turn-on, the walls would be decorated with pictures of Josef Stalin, Don Rickles, and an aerial view of East Berlin. To add to the lurid and erotic atmosphere, the customer would be given a heavy tweed overcoat to wear while the stereo blared out a medley of John Philip Sousa marches. The invigorating one-minute massage would be administered by two sumo wrestlers and the cost would be $100 per hour, plus tip. (I told you this was a sexy chapter.)

Owners of massage parlors and porno shops often use the Constitution as their defense, although we have no record of our founding fathers frequenting such establishments. The thought of the framers of the Constitution condoning such activity stretches the imagination. It is highly unlikely that *Poor Richard's Almanac* ever carried an ad that read: "Forging a new republic getting you down? Tonite, unwind at Madame Abigail's Colonial Casino of Carnal Cupidity." Is it possible that newspaper readers of the eighteenth century ever scanned such scurrilous hucksterism as: "Remember, all work and no play made Jack a dull forefather. This week, fly away to Benny's Bawdy Bunker Hill Penny Arcade. See a private live performance of *Love-Starved Maidens of Lexington and Concord.*"

What if the signers of the Declaration of Independence ever faced such enticements as: "Welcome, Continental Congress! Declare your independence at Sid's Sickie Book and Novelty Shoppe and pick up a copy of *Sensual Pleasures of the House of Burgesses.*"

Not even in the most run-down section of early Philadelphia was there ever a private, members-only club offering " '*Surrender at Yorktown*'—all male cast."

Or was there?

12. Privacy

Well, if you won't answer any of my census questions—would you like to buy a vacuum cleaner?

—LOCAL CENSUS TAKER

When the Census Bureau started warming up for the big head count of 1980, it was already clear that people were going to hold back on vital information. Therefore, the census takers had to sneak in the juicy questions among the bland ones to throw us off guard, such as: Name, age, and have you ever lusted after *a*) Howard Baker or *b*) pineapples? Have you ever had *a*) measles, *b*) smallpox, or *c*) relatives living in the Ukraine? What is your weight? What is your height? What is your astrological sign? What's your favorite movie? What's your favorite television show? What's your favorite illegal drug?

Favorite sports: (*check one*) *a*) pro football; *b*) other. If you checked *b* attach Form 12 to explain why.

Religion: *a*) Catholic; *b*) Protestant; *c*) Jewish; *d*) Druid; *e*) golf; *f*) tennis.

The next one is sneaky: Favorite color. Favorite hobbies. Do you wear artificial chest hair? If you are over forty, is your favorite holiday Halloween?

The reason this information was so important in 1980 was to give Uncle Sam the tools he needs to keep our commitment to the total invasion of privacy predicted for 1984.

Privacy no longer exists. In order to cope with its absence, we must change our attitudes and learn to love life in the fishbowl. My advice? Think positively, raise your window shades, gather your credit cards around you, and count your blessings.

Most people today are very concerned about threats to privacy by financial institutions, insurance and credit card companies, and so forth. Well, these people are paranoid, and they should send for

---

AND THAT REMINDS ME . . .

One hundred and two years after stealing land from the Sioux Indian nation, the United States government had to pay the tribe $100 million, which should give Japanese-Americans an idea bout how long they will have to wait for damages. The actual award was $17 million and the rest was interest.

The $17 million is the market value of the Black Hills region of South Dakota, the area in question. The government, in fact, may appeal, probably by attempting to prove that in 1877 the Indians were living in the South Bronx. We had a treaty with the Sioux and, reading between the lines, the treaty said: "You get the gravel and the weeds; we get the water, the oil, the gold, and the uranium. You get the sagebrush; we get the subdivisions and the shopping malls." So, with no deliberate speed, the tribe received its settlement.

A story like this always reminds me of one of those items about George Washington being made a five-star general retroactively, or Robert E. Lee eventually getting back his citizenship. The time of the Sioux incident occurred during the administration of General Ulysses S. Grant, who should at least one day be busted down to corporal.

Actually, the Indian should be grateful. We took his worthless grazing lands, green meadows, and clean water and turned it into the greatest interstate highway the world has ever known. Sure, the Indians could grow wheat and corn, but it was the white man who grew that miraculous hybrid—the concrete cloverleaf.

---

my book *Privacy Is for Hermits.* I try to show how to cope with your lack of privacy with such chapters as "Your Insurance Policy Number Is Your Friend" and "Talk to Your Credit Cards."

You see, the real reason why many people don't like giving personal information about themselves on applications is because they wish their lives were more exciting. For example, under "Occupation," instead of writing "clerk" they would rather write "middle linebacker." And under "Place of Birth," they wish they could put down Singapore instead of Duluth.

Lack of privacy can be a rewarding experience. If you lack privacy, flaunt it. Remember, your blood type brings you into a club with others of the same type. Are you a male, Protestant, Caucasian? Well, start feeling good about it. Your zip code is your neighborhood. Repeat after me: I pledge allegiance to my area code, and to the directory in which it stands; one color of eyes, indivisible, with annual income, and a social security number open to all.

13. For the Defense

Take my tanks—please!   —GENERAL HENNY YOUNGMAN

Take the high ground.   —GENERAL TIMOTHY LEARY

Take Ralph Nader.   —GENERAL MOTORS

First of all, you don't make fun of the military. You just don't do it. Goodness knows, there are enough things to lampoon, but the military is sacred. Better to knock something safe, like religion, than our soldier boys. They'll get you for it. Why risk the wrath of the American Legion, the Veterans of Foreign Wars, the Catholic War Veterans, the Jewish War Veterans, the Reformed Dutch Presbyterian War Veterans, and Barry Goldwater?

The song says, "I Love a Parade." Not, "I Hate a Parade." So when it passes by, cheer, don't sneer; otherwise someone might strike you on the noggin with a rock.

This is not to say that people in the armed forces don't have a sense of humor about themselves. They do—it's the ones on the fringe of military life who feel duty-bound to defend it when hardly necessary.

I was doing a radio show on a Sunday afternoon during a severe winter snowstorm in Washington in the mid-sixties. I was getting tired of reading the long list of school closings and other announcements radio people have to make on such a day, so I decided to break the monotony. I said, "Kindergartens in the area, along with the Humpty-Dumpty, Jack-and-The-Beanstalk, and Pixieland nursery schools will be open tomorrow—but the Pentagon will be closed."

No sooner had this innocent put-on fallen from my lips than the phone lit up.

"Who do you think you are, making fun of the Pentagon like that? You're un-American, that's what you are. You better make an apology because *my husband* works there!"

The Secretary of Defense didn't call, nor did I hear from the Chairman of the Joint Chiefs. No career officers or dedicated enlisted personnel took me to task for my impertinence, and no gung-ho top sergeant invited me outside to settle things. Only the lady whose husband worked at the Pentagon. And he was probably a civilian clerk typist.

A few years ago, I was doing a routine at the Shoreham about a scandal the Army was going through with their PXs. The top master sergeant in the entire army had been involved, along with other top-ranking personnel, in some kind of scheme that was not exactly in keeping with the ideals of General George Washington.

When I finished the show, I noticed a table of about a half dozen people in uniform. One of them was motioning for me to come over. As I walked to the table, I also noticed that they weren't smiling. One of them stood up, towering over me so that I felt like Mickey Rooney standing next to Wilt Chamberlain. Each ribbon, each commendation and oak leaf cluster adorning his barrel chest were like blinking road signs indicating danger ahead. The eagles on his shoulders looked alive and gave me a menacing look that made me feel as though Alfred Hitchcock had cast me in *The Birds*. His eyes darted out like laser beams from his John Wayne/George C. Scott face, and I just stood there wishing he would get it over with. The railroad spike that was his finger poked my chest like a jackhammer and he finally spoke: "You just keep on giving us hell whenever we need it."

Recently, however, one of the conclusions arrived at by a congressional committee investigating West Point in the wake of the academy's cheating scandals was that the school didn't have a sense of humor. Imagine an instructor at West Point conducting a joke-telling drill. A company of cadets standing in formation on the parade field shouts out in unison: "*A guy walks into a bar and sees a monkey behind the bar—Sir! He goes over to the piano player and says, 'Do you know there's a monkey behind the bar?'—Sir! And the piano player says, 'No, but if you'll hum a few bars maybe I can pick it out'—Sir!"*

Or perhaps some future MacArthur will recall this old barracks ballad of the 1970s:

WAR IS HELL

Now West Point is an institute of which we're very
    proud.
As a military academy, it's bloody but unbowed.
The only thing the students need that cannot be en-
    dowed,
Is: West Point doesn't have a sense of humor.

The students are ambitious, and the teachers never
    bores.
They spend their free time hazing plebes and doing
    other chores.
But if they want success, if they want bigger, better
    wars.
Then West Point better get a sense of humor.

The Pentagon has decided that Old West Point is a
    drag.
The students are too serious, so spirit starts to lag.
Now every underclassman must learn to tell a gag,
Because West Point doesn't have a sense of humor.

As a comic, I like Caesar, not Sid, but the guy from
    Rome.
And Hannibal and Alexander, they sent their writers
    home.
And don't you want to split a gut with Rommel, boy,
    he's some kind of nut!
But West Point doesn't have a sense of humor.

And when I think of Bill Westmoreland, he's a very
   funny guy.
His shtick is all together, as a comic rated high.
That "light at the end of the tunnel" line, I laugh until I
   cry!
But West Point doesn't have a sense of humor!

Now the most sublime comedians were Generals Grant
   and Lee,
Geniuses in all West Point history.
Why, Grant had such a sense of fun, he later proved the
   wrong man won.
But West Point doesn't have a sense of humor.

Now Custer was a general, a punster and a wit.
His one-liners all were formula, but somehow always
   fit.
His last words to the cavalry were "Boys, I guess the
   scalp's on me!"
But West Point doesn't have a sense of humor.

They're going to have new courses that will concen-
   trate on fun,
A seminar on custard pies, and Pratfalls 101.
They've got a course called "Ethnic Gag" and one on
   how to camp in drag
'Cause West Point's gonna get a sense of humor.

I think it's more than happenstance,
They've got a course called "Drop Your Pants."
And here's a course to blow your calm,
The name of it is "How to Bomb."

Now, Pershing had a funny walk, and Tojo had a tic.
Napoleon was a fruitcake, and Goering, he was sick.
Mountbatten and Montgomery, they were funny in a
   "funny" way!
But West Point better get a sense of humor.

When war finally destroys us, as it's prophesied to do.
And The Four Horsemen of the Apocalypse come rid-
      ing through.
The Army will be making jokes, like "tha-tha-that's all,
      folks,"
'Cause West Point went and got a sense of humor!

One of the more bizarre problems of having an all-volunteer army
was described by columnist Jack Anderson when he reported that
there were a number of card-carrying witches, practicing demons,
and Satan-worshipers in the military. A bewitching situation such
as this supported the theory that an army travels not on its stomach, but on its broom. Fort Dix will have to be changed to Fort
Hex, and Armed Forces Day will need to be switched to Halloween. It could be chaos in the mess hall as the time-honored army
tradition of griping brings about a new complaint: "Oh, no! Bat's
wings and lizard tongues on a shingle, again?"

    With witches in the Army, one can imagine the troops smartly
passing in review in their snappy uniforms, shined shoes, filed
teeth, and dead toads around their necks.

    The Anderson column went on to say that some military per-
sonnel were reported to be engaging in "festive ghost dancing in
the nude when the moon was full." That didn't surprise me because, if you were ever in the ranks, you'd recall that it was always
like that on pay day.

    I don't know how to deal with all of this. I suppose if we get rid
of the witches and demons, we'll have to go back to drafting students and pacifists.

    Of course, such G. I. skullduggery constitutes only a tiny mi-
nority of the military. On the other hand, a House subcommittee
under the chairmanship of Congressman Glenn English of Oklahoma determined that as many as one-third of our soldiers stationed in Germany are addicted to heroin and that possibly 70
percent use marijuana, hashish, and cocaine on a daily basis. And
since we have to make do with an all-volunteer army, which, it
would seem, is in no condition to fight, Madison Avenue, in order
to keep enlistments up, will have to launch a whole new kind of
advertising campaign:

"HEY BAAAAAABY! LOOKIN' FOR
A GOOD CONNECTION?"

(*Medium funk blues tempo*)

Let's get stoned and join the Army, that's the way to
  go.
I'm so wasted anyway, I can only feel one toe.
Sergeant says I got the duty, goin' on K.P.
You're on report for holdin' snort
If you don't give some to me.

Get some hash and join the action; that's the Army
  way.
Our smack gives you satisfaction every duty day.
Win service points for rollin' joints, no enemy to kill.
No M.P. squeals, 'cause the captain deals
That's my kind of G.I. Bill.

(*Fade music. Announcer up.*)

"Hi, out there, all you high school dropouts and losers.
Feel life is letting you down? Like to take drugs? Well,
look up an Army man and have him show you some
real hash marks. See your recruiter today and check it
out. Find out why A.W.O.L. stands for All Week Out
Laughin'. And hang loose—with Army green."

Philadelphia's former mayor Frank Rizzo once said on television
that his police department was tough enough to attack Cuba and
win. Wow! Today, Cuba; tomorrow, Washington. I'm worried,
since enlistments are down in all the branches of the service,
whether America can stand up to Philadelphia without reinstating
the draft? None of our eligible young people seem to have any interest in joining up, nor in the recruiting posters that say, "Join the
Army and see Philadelphia."

Once again, America is caught napping. While we've been fo-
cusing our attention on Russia, China and the Middle East, Philadelphia has been quietly building itself into a super-power. And

for all we know, they have their own air force tucked away some-place in New Jersey. So we must face the hard, cruel fact—Mr. Rizzo has got to be included in the SALT talks.

You notice that in our current relationship with Russia, no one mentions "détente" anymore. It's been a long time since politicians have used that word. That is because they have realized that détente is nothing more than going to a wife-swapping party and coming home alone.

You won't read about any of this in the "Humor in Uniform" department of *Reader's Digest*, nor in the magazine *Army Laffs*. The hawks tell us that this is what happens in a peacetime, all-volunteer situation. It's probably listed in some file in the Pentagon labeled "Peace, disadvantages of."

I suppose another of the disadvantages of peace would be that the longer it lasts, the fewer number of combat-experienced officers we'll have if war finally comes. Think of it—no officers will have won any higher decoration than the good conduct medal. They'll sit around the officer's club swapping such war stories as: "Did I ever tell you boys about the time I saw *The Longest Day* twice? There we were—as the Rainbow Division hit the beach at Normandy, I realized I was out of popcorn, so I surrendered my seat and made a tactical retreat to the lobby."

"Charlie, that reminds me of the time I was shopping for my wife in the commissary at Fort Bragg. To this day, I still break out into a cold sweat when I think about it. They were having a sale on cantaloupe and there were two left in the bin, see, and four other carts were closing in on them at two o'clock. Outnumbered, it was me against them. Just as I was making a direct approach toward the cantaloupes, I knew it was now or never. At the worst possible moment, the left front wheel on the cart jammed! I thought of bailing out but I just kept pushing. The cart started wobbling and shaking and going out of control. By now, I had forgotten about the cantaloupes, since I had all I could do to hold her steady. Just at that moment, the four enemy carts whizzed by me. So close that I could see the sneering faces of the people pushing them. That was my mistake. My cart plowed into a stacked pyramid of tomato juice cans six feet high. The sound was deafening—metal against metal—KABONG! KABONG! KABONG!—one can after an-other. It felt like a thousand of them falling on top of me, and I blacked out. When I came to, a crowd had circled around me, and I looked up and saw that the cantaloupe bin was empty. I still have this scar over my left eye. Eddie, give us another round, will ya?"

Such tales of glory will always fill our hearts with pride, and because of this aura of bravery and valor, the armed forces have an easier go of it than some of the other branches of government. For example, when it comes to a popularity contest, the Army, Navy, Marines, or Air Force always win over, say, the Department of Health, Education and Welfare. There is a reason for that—Hollywood never made a movie about a social worker. Politicians know that the easiest way to get a standing ovation when they are making a speech is to criticize the Department of HEW. Ridicule the Armed Forces, and they'll call you a left-wing, commie-pinko pervert. It's a plain fact that if the Secretary of Health, Education and Welfare wore a uniform with brass buttons and medals, she would get more respect.

Because of terrible public relations over the years, HEW has failed to capture the imagination of the American people. This is why it needs—a band! Oh, how our pulses have quickened to the stirring marches of our soldiers, sailors, and marines! How about some HEW marches: "From the Halls of Bedford-Styvesant," "Guidelines Aweigh," and "When the Welfare Checks Go Rolling Along."

For years, the glory of the military has been trumpeted through such great movies as *Sands of Iwo Jima, What Price Glory?* and *Patton.* A whole new way of public thinking could be brought about by producing some HEW motion picture classics: *Sands of a Lower-Income Neighborhood, What Price Social Security?* and the most stirring saga of blood and guts ever depicted on the screen, George C. Scott starring in *Nader.*

The opening scene of *Nader* is stupendous. The entire screen is filled with a 60-foot-high American flag, and a tiny figure appears at the bottom of the picture. Emerging forward, he soon appears larger than life and dominates the scene with his enormous presence. There is no doubt who he is—the pearl handled pistols of legend, 15 rows of ribbons, including the cross of Lorraine, the Croix de Guerre, the Legion of Merit, the Royal Order of the Seraphim, and the Grand Cordon of the Supreme Order of the Chrysanthemum—a red sash securing the sabre at the hip, standing firm in the leather puttees, and carrying a defiant swagger stick—none other than the fabled Nader himself.

He speaks. The gravelly voice gives the audience chills. "You people are here to become consumer advocates, dammit. One thing you must always remember is that no poor dumb bastard ever won a war against General Motors by dying for his country. The only way to win a war is by making the *other* poor dumb bastard die for *his* country. You gotta kick him in the ass—and you gotta go through him like crap through a goose!"

This same psychology has been worked upon our lawmakers for years, and the result has been ever-increasing defense appropriations. I'm not denying that the appropriations were warranted, but I am suggesting that the same psychology could be employed on behalf of other interests. Some of the persuasive tactics used by the Defense Department have been not only highly imaginative, but downright theatrical.

Everyone loves a show, and when you see a dazzling display of air power put on at an Air Force base, or stand on the bridge of an aircraft carrier as I have, and watch the exciting landings of the planes on the deck as they drop their hooks and catch the cable, you are sold on the entire program. (I've done some shows at the naval air station at Pensacola, Florida, and they once let me pilot the carrier U.S.S. *Lexington*. After I had taken the wheel, the captain said that, other than forgetting to use the turn signal, I did okay.)

When President Carter was treated to a massive mock battle costing $1 million staged for his benefit at Fort Hood, Texas, he wasn't about to go home to the White House and order the closing of Fort Hood. Nor should he have. But what about some equal spectaculars on behalf of social programs? I have in mind an outdoor super extravaganza, called "Hunger '80," or perhaps "Poverty Night Fever." Senators would receive a lasting impression as they observed, from the reviewing stand, a million starving people passing in review as the band played "Brother, Can You Spare a Dime?"

One of the rejected budget items several years ago was an appropriation for the removal of architectural barriers for the handicapped. The problem could have been emphasized by inviting our lawmakers to a wheelchair derby held at the Indianapolis speedway, with steps and revolving doors placed strategically along the track. These are all legitimate ways to capture the hearts and minds of our leaders, because there's no business like show business.

We seem to be neglecting the Navy here, so I'd like to tell you one of the great sea stories in the annals of naval history. The story took place at the submarine base in Groton, Connecticut, where they were assembling the 560-foot-long *Trident*, the granddaddy of all submarines.

This snappy runabout, longer than the Washington Monument, and weighing 18,700 tons, cost a billion dollars, not including FM radio and power windows. The Navy was rightly proud of this supreme sub, except for one thing—they couldn't get it to go underwater, at least not until they got it into the ocean. And the ocean was two and a half miles away. The river between the ocean and Groton, where they were building the *Trident*, was 36 feet deep. And the Trident had a water draft of—you're getting ahead of me—*36 feet, 6 inches.*

The outcome of the story is that the Navy did not give up the ship, but they did get rid of the five-dollar calculators.

For quite a while our defense posture was based upon the statistics of SALT I. I played around with the specifications of the arms limitation agreement and discovered that, under SALT, each side was limited to a figure of 1,320 multiple nuclear warheads—1,320 for the Russians, and 1,320 for us.

Now, just one of these warheads can completely wipe out a city. Even though there are not 1,320 Russian cities, I suppose we must be prepared in the event New Zealand or Monaco gets out of line. We'd have to slap them around a little bit—maybe just break their knees.

Do you realize that right at this very moment there's someone sitting at the Pentagon, 24 hours a day, whose job is to decide which 1,320 cities we want to blow up? Or maybe it's 660 cities we want to blow up twice? Or, come to think of it, the one city we want to blow up 1,320 times?

I've always been fascinated by government statistics—like the time the Air Force wanted 244 B-1 bombers. The reason they never got the B-1 had nothing to do with the plane at all; it was that confusing number. Why not 243, or 240, or round it out to an even 200? They were $100 million apiece, for godsake. Plus radio and heater! So President Carter canceled the B-1. The last time a president did away with a weapons system of that size was when Ulysses S. Grant told General Custer, "That oughta be enough ammo to hold you for a while."

The one most affected by the cancellation of the B-1 bomber was Rockwell International Corporation, because they were supposed to build it. After the B-1 was abandoned, the rumor was that Rockwell was in trouble and might have to merge with another company facing difficulty—the suit manufacturer Robert Hall. They would manufacture very cheap cruise missiles that do not fit.

The cruise missile was still a viable weapon, but again, the Air Force was confusing. Do you think they wanted an even 2,000? Wrong. They wanted 2,357. Where do they get these figures? How would those generals feel if their wives sent them to the store for 14 eggs?

Another item on our armament shopping list was the neutron bomb. As soon as the public was made aware of such a device, everyone imagined the neutron bomb to be just what the name implied— a bomb. But the military was quick to point out that this was not a Hiroshima mushroom-cloud-type thing, but rather an "enhanced radiation device" designed to kill people by radiation alone, leaving the buildings standing. The fact that it wouldn't have the characteristics of an atomic or hydrogen bomb was encouraging, since that, at last, meant we were going to do something about noise abatement. The idea of killing the humans but sparing the buildings was also intriguing. You could call it urban renewal for people. (Of course, another killer that wipes out people but leaves the buildings is the interest rates on home mortgages.) Dying by radiation alone has its drawbacks, however, since you could assume that this would keep the relatives away from the funeral. On the up side, it would mean increased sales for lead-lined coffins.

The neutron bomb planned for our NATO forces in Europe was designed primarily for use against Russian tanks. If a tank is coming at you, and you zap it with the enhanced radiation, you kill everybody inside. So what you have left is a tank running around aimlessly out of control. Doing what? Knocking down buildings. And there goes the neighborhood!

Well, we've talked about the Army, the Navy, and the Air Force, saving the best for last—those valiant warriors of the globe and anchor, the fabled leathernecks of song and legend, those glory happy devil dogs swaggering their way from the Halls of Montezuma to the shores of Iwo Jima, the proudest of the proud, the United States Marine Corps. I speak with authority now, because, yes, I was a marine. I became Private Marcus J. Ruslander-1380713 on March 19, 1953—a sad day for the corps. A day when the eagle climbed down from atop the globe to lie down and die. A date definitely not engraved in marble at the base of the Iwo Jima statue at Arlington.

Oh, sure, I could regale you with salty stories of my adventures in the corps—the night patrols, the skirmishes, the stinking foxholes, Pearl Harbor, Midway, Okinawa; but I'd rather not talk about it. Because I served in peacetime, that's why. I guess what I dread is the day when my children will come to me and ask, "What did you do in the peace, daddy?"

How impressed will they be if I tell the truth—that the only time I was in any real danger was during an inspection, when my sideburns were a half inch lower than the top of my ears. Regulations stated that "the sideburns will be trimmed to a level even with and not lower than the top curvature of the ear." For this infraction, the inspecting officer, noting that I looked like Fernando Lamas, gave me a week's restriction.

I don't know what it's like now, but the peacetime corps of the fifties was guided by one driving obsession—good grooming. Thinking that my days would be filled with weaponry and dangerous maneuvers, I enlisted, only to spend three years qualifying with the blitz cloth, brass polish, shoe polish, floor wax, and starch. Instead of coming home as John Wayne, I returned as Mr. Clean.

Most of my Marine Corps activity had to do, not with keeping the light of freedom burning, but with keeping my belt buckle shining. There simply was nothing else to do. It was the Marines' finest hour. Corps historians tell us that '53–'56 were their proudest years. The rifles were the cleanest, the shoes were at their highest state of gloss, you could dine on the hood of a jeep, every round of ammunition was neatly arranged in well-kept bunkers, tanks were show-room spotless, and bayonets were antiseptic and glittering. The corps had me to thank for all that.

When I see old films of World War II, I am appalled. Those men running up Mount Suribachi were filthy. Their uniforms were wrinkled and their boots were in a mighty sorry state, and I don't mind saying so. Sure, they raised the flag over Iwo Jima, but did you see the sideburns? A lot lower than the top of the ear, I'll tell *you.* That wasn't my Marine Corps, that's for sure.

In my corps, appearance counted for something. That's what I'll tell my sons: "Boys, you should have seen our floors. Your old Dad really knew how to run a buffer in those days. Why, when I got through cleaning windows, you didn't even know they were there. And Marines today don't even know what a collar stay is. No, sir. And their shoes are made out of that stuff that never needs shining. That's not the way it was when your dad was a Marine. Boys? Boys, wake up. I want to tell you about the wound I got when I cut myself on the crease in my pants. Nearly bled to death . . ."

14. How to Be a Father, and the Miracle of Birth—or— When You're Old, They Might Give You the Spare Bedroom

As a father, I never even came close to measuring up to Fred Mac-Murray. Fred and Robert Young and all the father figures of this century—Ike, Roosevelt, and Lewis Stone—have served as constant reminders of my paternal inadequacies. Compared to these all-time big-league fathers I never could shape up.

Take Fred MacMurray. Remember how, on "My Three Sons," whenever one of his kids had a problem, Fred was always perfectly composed in his den? As one of his sons poured out some grave disaster, like not having a date for the prom, which was four months away, Fred, always the perfect father, would sit at his desk, hands folded, in front of rows of books and offer words of wisdom: "Now son, there's still plenty of time and there's lots of fish in the sea. So run along and do your homework."

"Gee, thanks, Dad," said the lad as he skipped from the room. And Fred, puffing on his pipe would say, "Don't mention it, son."

For the rest of us out here in real life on the other side of the TV screen, it's never quite like that. In my case, whenever a family crisis develops, I am always in the bathroom, and you just can't offer advice and reason from in there. For one thing you never saw Fred shouting through a locked door. For another thing, there are no bookshelves in the bathroom, so what image of wisdom can you possibly portray as you sit there?

On Robert Young's show "Father Knows Best," he always did. Despite crisis upon crisis, one turmoil after another, fears were neatly put to rest as he stood in total command, wearing a tweed coat and tie and dispensing platitudes in front of the bookshelves.

Mickey Rooney always got into one mess after another in the old Andy Hardy movies. I was only about ten years old when they were being shown and what I remember most about them was his father, Judge Hardy, played by Lewis Stone. Judge Hardy, complete with vest and watch chain, shaped his son's destiny with ponderous intonations uttered at his desk in the library with row upon row of very serious-looking books looming directly behind him.

I have a desk and I have bookshelves but I'm never near them when there's trouble. When you are bumper to bumper in a hot holiday traffic jam in dire need of a gas station for multiple reasons, and one kid forcefully applies a toy truck to the side of the head of the other kid, causing shrieks and blood, where are those books when you need them? You don't have on a vest and watch chain to denote authority, and even if you did, they wouldn't go with your silly-looking Bermuda shorts.

I have thought about keeping a few books on hand in case of such emergencies wherever I go, as sort of a portable instant image-of-wisdom kit. For example, you're in a department store and your youngsters are pulling everything off the counters— "Buy me this!" "I want that!" You merely hold one of your books behind your head, for the desired effect, assume your best Fred MacMurray pose, and say, "Now, son, put that back. Remember, a penny saved is a penny earned. Squander not, my boy, and heed the value of thrift!" Sure, you might get a few stares, but then so did Fred.

Finally, the kids get old enough to start life on their own. They've reached a certain maturity, and you think the hard years of being a parent are behind you. Well, you think wrong, because the hard years are never behind you; there are always more just ahead.

It is said that when a young bird is about to leave the nest it begins craning its neck and twitching its wings. At that moment, the mother bird knows that her cuddly pride and joy has tired of the old homestead and is soon to fly off to meet life's adventures. With a human offspring in her late teens, the signals of the impending fleeing of the coop differ from craning and twitching. Perhaps you've spotted the clue with your daughter already: it's when you say just about anything at all to her, and the answer is, "I knew you were going to say that." Now it's true that we said "I knew you were going to say that" to our parents, but that was different. Perhaps it's an embarrassment to hear it because when we say what they knew we were going to say, *we* think it to be a pearl of great wisdom and expect the daughter to reply, "Dad, your knowledge amazes me. Thanks for the insight. I'm going to have to remember that." Instead, loving advice such as "Pizza and root beer isn't the best breakfast, sweetheart," or "Your friend who got married in the ninth grade might be missing a bit in life," is greeted with "I knew you were going to say that."

My advice? When you've made your profound statement, tell them: "I know what you're going to say."

Perhaps you can identify with the following scene:
We walk down a corridor and enter a suite of rooms that is an

interior decorator's dream. The graceful draperies blend harmoniously with the lush carpet, which accentuates the impeccable design of tasteful furniture. The accessories are lively but understated: the pictures on the wall superb reproductions; each pillow a plump delight; each plant a lovely poem. Stereophonic music plays the classics in an eloquent testimony to the flawless taste of the inhabitants.

Where are we? The presidential suite at the Waldorf? No, but you're close. The queen's bedroom at Buckingham Palace? Not quite. We are standing in a girl's dormitory in any university in America. Perhaps I exaggerate slightly, but as the parent of a college freshman, I feel that anyone in the carpet, stereo, drapery, or plant business is crazy unless he has an outlet near a college.

At the same time, over in the boy's dorm, they are doing a continuous performance of *Animal House*, live. In a recent report, the average college male student at an eastern university drinks 87 gallons of beer per term. When they talk about the Spring Hop, they don't mean Saturday night's dance.

If the kids don't give you a hard time, count on the government to make it tough to be a parent. A few years ago someone at HEW said that father and son nights were illegal because they exclude women. This ruling frightened me into coming out into the open. Acting on the advice of my lawyer that I had attended an illegal father and son night, I pleaded *nolo contendere*, and signed an affidavit saying that the clandestine meeting was held in a hidden bunker under the gymnasium floor of my son's school. Pouring out my confession, I described further details of the illegal act. My hands still shake as I write this, but while the fathers and sons played games, sang songs, and drank root beer, lookouts were stationed at the entrance watching for any agents from the Anti-Father and Son Task Force of HEW.

Before going to the meeting, I had instructed my son that if we were arrested, "Tell them I'm your mother."

A few weeks later, a friend of mine told me that his wife and daughter went to a mother and daughter night and he hadn't heard from them since. He assumes they have been arrested and are being held incommunicado until one agrees to a sex-change operation.

All this stress and strain in being a parent can age you. And old age is not exactly something to look forward to.

As soon as people begin acquiring the genuine wisdom that comes only with age, we retire them. Only recently, we have begun to attack the mandatory retirement age, which is bad news for the gold watch industry.

Next on the list should be the elimination of ageist stereotypes, such as "little old ladies." How come you never hear of big old ladies? Or, for that matter, dirty young men?

I never felt any real pangs about growing older until October 17, 1977. That was the day I read that Ricky Nelson was 36. I probably would have been better off not knowing that depressing little fact. It brings on the same feeling that comes when your children tell you they are learning about Lyndon Johnson in history class.

Another little tell-tale sign of aging is the suspicion that the people who print the phone book are engaged in a conspiracy to get you into bifocals. Bifocals, we always thought, were only for those people in the audience who dance on the Lawrence Welk show.

Whether to be a parent at all in the United States can be examined from two different perspectives. From one point of view, we are having too many babies; from another, we aren't producing enough. The Supreme Court decision legalizing abortions immediately transformed the subject into a political issue. The position I took was that those favoring abortion were people who had already been born. The candidates in their typical fashion usually attempted to please all sides at once. In 1976, Jerry Ford seemed to be saying, "I'm against abortion—except in states with major primaries."

Several years ago, I suggested the only practical solution to the abortion controversy but nobody would listen. My idea was federal tax credits for vasectomies—but only if accompanied by a swine flu shot.

The real complications arose when Congress began dealing with the subject. As I understand it, the House ruled that a woman may receive federal funds for an abortion up to and including the eleventh day of pregnancy, providing she was examined by two doctors, a senator, and the Speaker of the House.

When the anti-Equal Rights Amendment people held a victory celebration in Washington, it appeared to be quite different from the rallies we usually see around here. I remember the tear gas and marijuana of the anti-war marchers, shouts of "Hell, no, we won't go!," the racial disturbances in 1968, and the farmers digging up the place on occasion. But the anti-ERA crowd is composed of homemakers, who having just fixed dinner for their hubbies, did the dishes and then popped down to Washington demanding the right to be prim.

Their leader, Phyllis Schlafly, who could be played by Jane Wyatt, the actress who played the wife on "Father Knows Best," attacked the liberals by telling a Chappaquiddick joke. Well, one lady laughed so hard she almost fell off her pedestal. Yes, once they get out of the kitchen these finalists in the Pillsbury Bake-Off can be just as strident as their feminist foes. And a demonstration by either crowd can drive you out of the house and down to the corner bar for a drink with the boys. As I left the rally the ladies were dusting the furniture in the hotel lobby, chanting their anti-ERA slogans, "Dinner's ready, honey," "Oh, goody! I'm pregnant," "The car won't start, it must be the thing-a-ma-bob," and "Fiddledy-dee, fiddledy-dee, we don't want an IUD!"

I mentioned the point of view that we were not producing enough babies. This was an opinion expressed by a doctor at Princeton University who said that we Americans were getting so good at birth control that the government may have to start paying people in the future to maintain the population.

The Federal Procreation Program I visualize makes great use of slogans for propaganda purposes, such as "Uncle Sam Wants You to Get Careless," "Pregnancy Is Patriotic," and "Eight Is Not Necessarily Enough." Under the program, a couple notifies the newly formed Department of Multiplication that an attempt to have a baby has been made. The DOM sends the couple one multiplication stamp for each attempt. The stamps are stuck into a special book, and when the book is filled it may be taken to a multiplication redemption center in exchange for a cash prize. Or the couple may decide to save a number of filled books (plenty of incentive here). The more books, the better the prizes—toasters, miocrowave ovens, golf clubs, and so on.

I suppose a discussion of birth in these advanced technological times should include its more bizarre aspects. I'm thinking of test-tube babies, specifically the one born in England in the summer of 1978. At that time it was clear that Great Britain had become Mediocre Britain, and that it did not have its old class or dignity. The British can be just as tacky as the rest of us, as we noted in the behavior of the British press regarding the birth of the little girl, conceived outside the mother's womb. It's safe to predict that the child will enjoy the normal life accorded to the Dionne quintuplets and the respected privacy enjoyed by the Lindberghs.

The *London Daily Mail*, which can make any American scandal magazine look like the Congressional Record, paid half a million dollars for the exclusive serialization of the child's historic entry into the world. And get this: if the baby failed to live a week, the newspaper's subscribers would get 40% off. If the baby failed to live 28 days, another big cash refund. And the newspapers were notified that these rights were for the first 400 days of the child's life.

Did anybody believe they'd stop there? When the Dionne quintuplets were well into their 30s, the press was still at it. And who doubts that the day will come when we'll see a caption, "Test-tube baby goes to the prom."

I can see the ad now. "Yes, only in the *Daily Mail* can you get news, sports, weather, the late-breaking baby results, plus the name-the-sex-lottery, the baby crossword, the goo-goo gossip column, and the coupon for your very own test tube-key charm."

Science has also brought about a solution for those who believe there should be more people in the world exactly like themselves. Cloning, or the do-it-yourself self, poses the possibility of creating an organism from a body cell outside the normal process of conception—although not as much fun. In other words, if an embryo were to be created from you alone, it wouldn't be your child, it would be you! A genetically identical duplicate of yourself. Think of it—Xeroxed people!

When the cloning stories first appeared, I feared for the future.

What if someone should write a song called "I Want a Girl Just Like the Girl Cloned from Dear Old Mom." I also worried about what would happen when these little clones grew up and had to fill out simple forms. After "Father?" what would they write, "Me"?

Where would an Annual Clone Convention be held—the Twin Cities? Walla Walla? Baden Baden? Would they work to fight clone discrimination? How would people react if a clone moved in next door? How would they know whether the clone might have lived there all along as his original self?

Sure it's weird and freaky, but then isn't this country great because of self-made men? And let's not forget the fathers who are coping with M.L.C. (Mid-Life Crisis), the ones who dress a little younger with every passing year.

Let's make every day Father's Day. Sit the gray-haired swinger in his easy chair, fetch him his hash pipe and sandals, and sing that old favorite, "I Want Some Beads Just Like the Beads That Hang on Dear Old Dad."

Am I imagining, strange things are happening, and changing dear old Dad?
We don't know the cause. Mom says it's male menopause, or just some passing fad.
Last week, for example, he traded in the car for a lobster-red Ferrari, then went out and bought a singles bar.
Each day's a new surprise, he's thrown out his coats and ties,
We hardly know old dad.

To the office he wears turquoise beads, eats yogurt and sunflower seeds, Dad sure is acting weird.
Last month he grew a beard, and his ponytail looks great.
It seems a strange pursuit, free falling in a parachute, when he's nearing forty-eight.
According to statistics he is not alone
Once he read the *Wall Street Journal,* now it's *Rolling Stone.*

His old self is what he loathes, while wearing those
    teenage clothes,
There's a change in dear old Dad.

According to the experts behavior like this tells
That he wants to be Burt Reynolds, but he's built like
    Orson Welles.
Old Dad's sure in a bind, trying to keep young in mind,
But we love him, dear old Dad.

15. Joy of Tax

If, as a result of our preparing your return, you must
pay more tax than you thought you would, we will
gladly pay for the stamp and the envelope.

—H&R CROCK

Since there is no reason why people can't get more satisfaction out
of paying taxes than they do, I have prepared a book, complete
with stimulating pictures, on achieving pleasure with the Internal
Revenue Service. In my new book, *Joy of Tax,* I discuss everything you've always wanted to know about it, but were always
afraid to ask. The word "tax" seems to frighten some people, and I
think it's because when most of us were children, they didn't have
tax education in the schools. We had to pick it up on the street corner. Your father probably took you off behind the barn to explain
where dependents came from, but today, with the breakdown of
old taboos, people are more willing to discuss their tax lives freely.
Some, worrying about being overtaxed, decided to cut back. They
are called Californians. And for years, people overdid it when it
came to imposing their sometimes weird tax practices on others.
They were called liberals. But a good, healthy tax life with someone you love can bring joy and fulfillment. But it means caring and
sharing. It means communicating, especially on April 15.

For some time, members of Congress expressed a desire to vote themselves a $50-a-day income tax deduction to cover the cost of keeping two homes. I think they deserve the relief, but the money should come from the private sector. How? By legalizing bribery. I agree that Congress needs a break, but this is what happens when you treat Tongsun Park so shabbily that he cuts off your cash flow.

In order to gain public support for giving themselves a tax break, senators should do television commercials, like the one for Geritol. The senator looks right into the camera and says, "After working all day for others, I take a tax break every day. It's just a little something I do for myself." Then the senator's wife walks into the picture, puts a reassuring arm around his shoulder, and says, "This is my husband and he takes real good care of himself. I think I'll keep him."

Members of Congress now make $60,700 a year, and it's necessary for them to maintain two houses. But what about the man with one house who makes only half as much as a congressman, or $30,350 a year? If senators want a $50-a-day break, shouldn't the guy making $30,350.00 get a $25-a-day deduction?

And so in these days of austerity, cutting the budget, and trimming the fat, as Congress prepares to help themselves to a $2.5 million a year from the treasury, let the rest of us be soothed by the words of Jimmy Carter, who once said, "Life is unfair."

Now, children, I'll tell you a story of the IRS Form 949, the little form that couldn't. You've probably never heard of Form 949. It's not one of your big name forms, like 1040 or the famous W-2. Ten-forty and W-2 get all the publicity and attention at the Internal Revenue Service. Ten-forty gets printed by the millions and goes into every home. The poor little 949 never had a chance at that kind of audience.

Nine-four-nine was supposed to go to corporations. It was the profit control form to be sent to contractors selling ships and planes to the Pentagon. Under the law, strict limits are set on profits made on these sales. In 1979 Form 949 was to have been sent to these corporations by April 15, but the poor little form never got off the ground. You know why? The IRS never got around to printing it, and then said that it would take six months to do so. By then the Pentagon could lobby the defenseless form out of existence. And, so, once again, Big 1040 won, and corporations were left uncontrolled. Individuals get all the breaks.

Everyone knows that if you divorce your spouse and continue to live together, you get a big tax break. It's as if the government asks, "As a hedge against inflation, for the sake of the children and family unity, have you considered divorce?"

There has been opposition to these laws, which say that if a man and his working wife earn $40,000 and get divorced, they could save over $1600 in taxes every year. Just about enough to pay for an uncontested divorce, and then it's all gravy. The tax folks love this law because it would cost $4.8 billion a year to change it. Constitutionalists love it because it reaffirms the separation of church and state. In other words, a sin is not a crime.

Ah, to hear the sound of laughter and the clinking of champagne glasses in the divorce court. The happy couple no longer married, beaming fondly as their friends toss handfuls of stove-top stuffing mix at them and the band plays "The Second Time Around" and "One Alone." Then everyone throws confetti, made from old 1040 forms run through a shredder. Finally, we see the divorced couple driving off together with single-serving soup cans tied to the bumper.

The Supreme Court has decided that divorced husbands do not have to pay alimony if their ex-wives are making more than they are. I guess, among other things, this means that Elizabeth Taylor will finally have to let Eddie Fisher off the hook.

Obviously, the Supreme Court knows that it's just not right when the wife gets to keep the Renoir, the Steinway, and the beach house, and the husband gets to keep the '49 Studebaker. Then he has to sell it to make his alimony, and she cashes the check at the El Swanko Hacienda in the Bahamas.

The next thing the Court should do is take up visitation rights. I say it's time for the mothers to take the kids to the zoo on the first Sunday of the month. Let's redistribute the guilt around here, and let the mother shower presents on the kids for a change and take them on trips. If it weren't for divorce, there'd be no Disneyland.

Alimony can be very inhibiting. I know a divorced man who was so henpecked when he was married, he now stays five months ahead on his payments. Thank goodness the court has struck down

AND THAT REMINDS ME . . .

I ask you, what can compare to the joy of watching little kittens frolicking on a freshly mown lawn, or a sunset on a summer's eve, or a casino in New Jersey getting its license?

Exactly one year before the ABSCAM scandal, the New Jersey Casino Control Commission granted a license to Resorts International, finding "no evidence of organized crime involvement in that company." There were pictures in the paper of people cheering and embracing each other, and I must confess that I wept when I saw them. I always cry at exorcisms. Can't you see it now: The high commissioner standing among the craps tables; he raises his arms and cries, "Away, away, ye vile and wretched devils of organized crime. I declare this place to be pure." The gamblers drop to their knees, weep tears of joy, look up to the high commissioner, and cry out, "He has washed away the evil syndicate from gambling. Truly a miracle! Oh, rue the day when Resorts International's shares were less than a dollar—and now 50 and a quarter, up 7 points from Friday's close. All praise to the great gods Baccarat and Keno!"

Yes, in a sometimes dark and wretched life, we know there is a better world—and it is called New Jersey. Just follow the yellow brick turnpike and watch for the signs to Atlantic City.

these archaic laws, including the one that requires a man behind in his alimony to wear a dead duck around his neck.

Although they needn't be, taxes are a bugaboo to most people. I trust the reader will find peace and contentment in these suggestions of what to do if you are audited.

1. Don't panic. The examiners want to be helpful. Usually they'll try to locate a prison near your family.
2. Bring your receipts with you. If you don't have them all, borrow some from a neighbor.
3. Answer questions truthfully. Before going to the audit practice your answers in front of a mirror without giggling. Chances are you already know what the questions will be.
4. Remember, the professional who prepared your crooked return

will go to the audit with you. Not as a legal representative, mind you, but to supply the Kleenex.

5. Do not—repeat—*do not* open the conversation by asking the examiner if he'd like an all-expense-paid trip to Acapulco.
6. Keep in mind that if the IRS itself helped you with your return, which later was found to be incorrect, they are not responsible. Either pay the money you owe or suddenly begin a new life as a citizen of the nearest nation without extradition rights.

Whenever we approach the income tax deadline the best thing to do is relax. Paying taxes is a patriotic duty. So be positive, be optimistic, be confident, and start thinking about what you'll wear to the audit. A Congressional Medal of Honor wouldn't hurt.

16. Thought for Food—or— Eat Your Fiber Cereal Before It Shrinks

Pass the potatoes.   —JOHN BELUSHI

I have always had this theory that there are benefits of food other than nutritional: religious (Fill my belly and I'll listen about your god); political (Let them eat cake); and musical (Yes, we have no bananas). Finally there's the appearance of food. Every artist in history, immortal and amateur, painted at least one bowl of fruit, because they knew that apples and pears looked nicer than door knobs and street scenes of Gary, Indiana.

Jokes with food in them seem funnier, even though the food may not even be relevant to the punch line. Perhaps our brains salivate like our taste buds, and when food is mentioned, we anticipate an ending of a joke to be funnier than it actually turns out to be.

Therefore, such stories render us more receptive. For example: "A guy walks into a restaurant and the waiter says . . ." or "What did the mayonnaise say to the refrigerator?" or "As the Idaho potato said to his daughter, 'I will not allow you to marry Dan Rather. He's just a common tater'."

Before our food is eaten by the consumer, it must first be grown by the farmer and then regulated by the Federal Trade Commission. This regulatory agency oversees groceries, transportation, and funeral directors. Hence its initials, FTC, which really stand for Food, Trucks, and Coffins.

The particular food most associated with the FTC is cereal. Every so often, there is an attempt to ban sugar-coated cereal commercials on children's television shows. If the ban ever came about, one advantage would be that kids wouldn't want to watch TV and we would all get some sleep on Saturday mornings. Another way to look at it would be that Saturday morning thrives on sugared products. Before they were marketed, there were only six and a half days in the week.

The FTC's ban won't work because its members simply do not know kids. Boys and girls will get that stuff into their bodies, TV or no TV, because each child has a secret connection. This connection, whose code name is Mom, will always deliver the stuff. All the kid has to say is, "Get some Sweeties, the all-new sugar-coated sugar with sugar topping—huh, Mom?" Sweeties, of course, are nothing but pure sugar—you pour it into a bowl and add corn flakes. (Just once, I'd like to see a Saturday morning show sponsored by creamed chipped beef on toast, the breakfast of Army brats.)

Here's how the connection makes the drop. Mom goes and makes the purchase and delivers it to the kid because she knows it will make him happy. It should. Even the kid is presweetened. Once he's had his fix, he's content. He knows what he wants and how to get it. He's smart. Smarter than the Federal Trade Commission.

The FTC wants to print labels warning of the dangers of eating too much sugar. (They should put a label on Mom that says sometimes *she* is too sweet and dangerous to her kids' health.) The label I picture on the cereal boxes is one that says, "Warning: Failure to eat this cereal can be harmful to the profits of Kellogg, Quaker, and

General Mills." It seems that the cereal manufacturers can pre-sweeten anything but the FTC. I suppose the way to do that would be to come out with a special cereal just for them—*Regulaties.*

The Saturday morning announcer would make the pitch in the middle of "Scooby Doo": "Ya know, gang, to be a winner on the Federal Trade Commission, you've got to be in top shape. And that means a good nutritious breakfast of *Regulaties*—the breakfast of champion Federal Trade Commissioners. If you want to score, whether on the commission or in private practice, start your day with *Regulaties.*"

Television not only convinces kids that sugary cereals are good for them, but it has many grownups believing that Will Rogers ate Grape Nuts. The commercials for Grape Nuts, done by Rogers's son, Will Rogers, Jr., bring up the following point: If the FTC succeeds in taking children's cereal commercials off the air because the cereals might not be good for them, shouldn't they force the makers of Grape Nuts to prove that their product will turn you into a beloved cowboy humorist? Or that if you purchase a certain perfume for Christmas, your wife will start looking like Catherine Deneuve? Or that if you give a particular brand of after-shave lotion to your husband, he will turn into Joe Namath? There is no difference between children and adults in the mind of Madison Avenue. We are all gullible defenseless ninnies.

But getting back to Will Rogers. Maybe as Will Jr. keeps telling us, his Dad really did eat Grape Nuts. Does that mean that the actor James Whitmore eats imitation Grape Nuts?

Frankly, a lot of marketing techniques confuse me. I never could understand a promotion gimmick once used by some supermarket chains, which involved the selling of classical record albums. With a certain amount of groceries, the shopper received a coupon. With enough coupons, the shopper would receive a classical album. Some stores have done the same thing with encyclopedias. Now I like classical music very much, but I think this practice is unfair, unless it would be possible to go into a record store and pick up a pint of cottage cheese. That also goes for motor oil, antifreeze, oil filters, and fan belts, which are, but shouldn't be, found in grocery stores.

The record deal that featured ads for a sale on broccoli, beans, and Brahms presented some problems. Consider the man with all nine Beethoven symphonies standing in the eight-packages-or-less express line. How embarrassing when the clerk says, "Sir, you're going to have to put one of those symphonies back." While the promotion was going on, I overheard a lady in the supermarket ask if the Faust was fresh, and at another point, a very angry customer demanded his money back. He threw the albums on the counter and snarled, "This Schubert symphony isn't finished."

Big, modern, one-stop supermarkets are handy. But the food that cost $10 four years ago costs $14.65 today. And at least, ten years ago, potato chips didn't come in a can. And $30 worth of food didn't fit into the glove compartment. Too bad we can't eat the fifty cents' worth of plastic and styrofoam that comes with a pound of hamburger. Just yesterday, a panhandler stopped me on the street and said, "Hey buddy, can you spare twenty-five dollars for a Mister Coffee?"

Shoppers have learned that the best time to lay in a supply of food is just before an election, since after the election the prices always go up. For years the prevailing rumor was that food prices were going up 7 to 10 percent. Now it's much more. When you consider President Carter's 8 percent guidelines, this puts you in such a hole that you often don't have hamburger to add to the helper. As a result, people either started using recipes from Julia Child's book *Gourmet Scraps* (Ham Hocks Lorraine, Hash Tartare), or else just lined up in the store to view the priceless Hope Cutlet. When you finally tired of Colonel Sanders' latest—Kentucky Fried Tripe—you could cut down on meat by seeking out a fanatic vegetarian, since nothing promotes dieting as much as listening to someone speak of animal cadavers or the glories of a rutabaga steak.

Although some of the food chains have come out with brand-X, no-frills items that cost anywhere from 15 to 30 percent less, buying them meant that I would have to say good-by to many of my old friends. These foods don't carry a label such as "Mother Fletcher's Succulent Home Grown Farm Fresh Sweet-Tasting Green Beans." No, the label on them simply says, "Green Beans." At the very least, they could have a government-inspired label like that in the Army which said, "Beans, green, Model M-1."

These non-brand-name items sounded like a good idea at first. The food was supposed to be just as nourishing, but I missed those tempting labels. I shuddered at the thought of breakfast without the spectacle of the pole vaulter or the basketball star in live action, leaping out at me from the box of Wheaties. What would peanut butter taste like without Mr. Peanut winking at me every morning? My mind was made up: buying the no-frills food was not worth saying good-by to old friends like Aunt Jemima and Uncle Ben. Why, they practically raised me as a boy. I've grown older, but they're just as spry as ever. And the little girl spilling the salt on the ground—she never got home. She's been walking for 30 years or more. I can't leave her now. For a few cents more it's worth it to visit with the smiling Quaker man, Mrs. Butterworth, the Pillsbury Dough Boy, and the Jolly Green Giant. Because nobody likes to eat alone.

But what really counts are the basics of food itself. The miracle of the tiny seedling creates a new life. A new life brings nourishment to the planet as the earth replenishes itself. And what is more emblematic of our nation than amber waves of grain? And man took those grains and pounded them into flour and created a staple, a staple that is the essence of America—lasagne!

From farmer to farmer, from parent to child, another great American tradition is passed down to each generation—make the prairies bloom unless the government pays you not to.

I don't understand the politics of agriculture, but I do enjoy food; therefore I'm for the farmer. Everytime the farmers come rumbling into Washington with those big tractors, I try to learn. When they threatened to go on strike, I believed them, although as a city dweller I couldn't understand how a farmer would strike. I could understand steel workers or longshoremen walking off the job, but how does a farmer do it? Does he stop the milking and let the cows blow up? Does he picket his own fields and chant, "Hell, no, we won't grow?"

There is always considerable confusion and limited patience when the farmers come to town, due to the clogging of the traffic by the tractors. The government workers, held up in traffic, have a hard time getting to work, which is exactly what the demonstrating farmers had in mind. What eventually is going to happen, I believe, is that the federal employees will strike back at the farmers for the inconvenience. They will retaliate by driving a bureaucratic caravan of limousines into downtown Wichita, Kansas, and litter the streets with twists of lemon and empty gin bottles.

Which brings up the three-martini lunch. Jimmy Carter once had the audacity to suggest that this cherished tax deduction be abolished. Presidents have been brought up on impeachment charges for less treasonable offenses. Lunch is what turns the wheels of democracy and the stomachs of the mighty. Everything right or wrong about our country comes about when a person looks another squarely over the left shoulder and says, "Let's have lunch."

The possibility of the end of the tax-deductible business lunch moved me to form an environmental organization along the lines of Save the Whales or Save the Redwoods. My cause was Save Lunch or Business Stops (SLOBS).

Lunch is what makes America work—even waiters, bartenders, and waitresses. Consider what would happen without the business lunch. Executives having nowhere to go for three hours a day would roam the streets. Since no more business would ever be transacted again, millions of attaché cases would contain only tuna fish salad sandwiches. If you think we've got unemployment now, wait until all those distilleries close down. Swank restaurants would be forced to limit their menus to two choices—the barrel or the bucket.

The three-martini lunch, being only a euphemism for the deductible meal with two to four participants, would also include deductible banquets and other corporate extravaganzas, such as convention entertainment. Which means that with a change in the tax structure concerning business-oriented dining, the main night club at a Las Vegas hotel could feature only one strolling accordionist.

Whenever our lawmakers turn their attention to food and hold hearings on the subject, the hearings are well attended. I suppose it's because they are a welcome departure from global doom, corruption, and OPEC nose thumbing. Some time ago Congress took a look at the fast food franchises, and all the chicken and hamburger superstars came to Capitol Hill to testify—Roy Rogers, Minnie Pearl, Joe Namath, Mahalia Jackson, and a substitute for Johnny Carson.

In the case of Namath, Jackson, and Carson, their restaurants never caught on, which is what the hearings were all about. Carson went to men's suits, Namath went to pantyhose, and Mahalia Jackson went to heaven.

The hearings also revealed that an investor in a restaurant bearing a celebrity's name is gambling on that star's popularity. Show biz being what it is, you could be on top one day and on the bottom the next. I should know, since I once bought stock in Sonny Tufts' Baloney Sandwiches, Morey Amsterdam's Maison de Crêpes, Colonel Henny Youngman's Down Home Bar-B-Que, and Yvonne DeCarlo's Frozen Yogurt.

One restaurant that I have purposely left out of this discussion is Arthur Treacher's Fish & Chips. Oh, there's nothing wrong with the food, it's just that I knew the courtly Britisher, and I always had great difficulty picturing him in any roadside quickie food outlet, his own or otherwise. There is something sacrilegious about a picture of this distinguished stage veteran hoisted over our nation's highways with the Midas Muffler signs, Radio Shack, Tastee Freeze, Dairy Queen, and, heaven help us, Jack-in-the-Box. Arthur Treacher dined at Sardi's and "21," and to make him a fixture on every drag strip in middle America is the same as sentencing Robert Morley to ten years of flying economy class on Inter-Gulch Airways ("Our planes stop where you are—cleared runway or not!").

George McGovern, of all people, got into the fast food business; not on the highway ("Colonel McGovern's Dakota-Fried Steak"), but on Capitol Hill. The senator headed a subcommittee that, having conducted an investigation, defended the nutritional value of McDonald's hamburgers and Kentucky Fried Chicken. Perhaps McGovern had no choice, because they took away his reservation at the Sans Souci after he lost his bid for the presidency.

I suspect that the reason politicians don't eat in fast food restaurants is because they don't have tablecloths to pass the money under. Come to think of it, the last time I saw a senator at McDonald's he was sending back the root beer complaining about the bouquet.

The hamburgers had been sent to McGovern's hearing room by Ronald McDonald. The clown, lonely for the circus life, visited Capitol Hill and was immediately surrounded by dozens of gleeful, screaming youngsters jumping up and down—most of whom were freshmen members of Congress.

So, George McGovern, United States senator, presidential candidate, and great American, received the thanks of a grateful nation, having presided over these difficult hearings day after day, eating Big Macs, Quarter Pounders with Fries, the bucket and the barrel, regular and extra crispy, all of which he pronounced to be *cuisine magnifique.* After the hearings, a solemn-faced McGovern faced a battery of reporters and said, "I pardoned Colonel Sanders because he has suffered enough."

Then there was the time the government moved to ban snack (junk) foods in most schools, "until after lunch is served." What the government doesn't know is that lunch itself is pizza, Sloppy Joes, Burritos, and carbonated imitation raspberry-flavored drink mix.

After years of research, the Department of Agriculture finally succeeded in defining junk food. I always wondered, if they didn't know what it was, why didn't they ask us?

You don't think I'm going to attack junk food? Not by your Cheese Doodle I'm not! Attack the very foundations of this Republic—Mom, the flag, and barbecue-flavored potato chips? And risk an investigation by the FBI? Think again, my friend. Junk food is what makes America work. It's what we decorate the landscape with. I ask you, what would the median strips of our nation's highways be without ice cream wrappers, half-eaten Hardeeburgers, Schlitz empties, miles of styrofoam cups, wrappers, and containers from sea to shining sea? Those median strips would be nothing but monotonous acres of grass, bushes, and trees, that's what.

The government, by attempting to slow down the sale of candy, chewing gum, frozen desserts, sodas, and foods having less than the minimum daily requirement of protein, niacin, and thiamin, is biting off more than it can chew, because any official who thinks a kid will eat an apple instead of a bag of cheese munchies doesn't have any children at home under the age of 27.

17. What Now, Know-How?

Mr. Watson, I want you! —ALEXANDER GRAHAM BELL

The number you dialed is not in service. —MR. WATSON

Whenever I grow weary of the quest for mirth in the legislative process, I turn to the latest news from the world of technology. I approach the subject with a pure and innocent heart, not only uncomprehending of the computer, the laser, and the optic fiber, but also the pencil sharpener, the bicycle brake, and the cab meter.

Thank goodness there is at least one nation that has the stick-to-it savvy to use its technology for bringing about a higher standard of living. Let's hear it for the same pioneer spirit that gave us the automobile, television, and the microwave oven. Let's hear it for Japan.

Our relationship with Japan has changed because we now buy their sophisticated electronics and they buy our firecrackers and paper umbrellas. There is a reason for this. Once President Carter asked Emperor Hirohito what the secret of Japan's enormous success was, and the emperor was heard to reply, "Well, you Americans have already lost one war; so you're on the right track." The two leaders seemed to get along fine, and Hirohito offered to let his pilot fly Carter on a sightseeing trip around Japan. Carter thought it was a great idea until he learned that Hirohito's pilot never learned to land. While the president's party was in Japan, the entertainment for them featured a showing of the Gregory Peck movie *MacArthur*, which was run backward so that Japan wins.

The president had mentioned that on the way home he had planned to stop off in Hawaii for a private vacation. Hirohito suggested that the best way to go was to fly there early Sunday morning, before anyone was up.

A commentary on the times we live in is that one of the most fascinating news stories of the past several years dealt with the possibility of a giant orbital space station plunging out of control toward Earth, perhaps to crash into the middle of a city.

Skylab, when launched in 1973, was unnoticed by the general public, which was preoccupied at the time with the daily bombshells of Watergate. Six years later, however, when the spacecraft slipped its orbit, America held its breath and sang (who says we can't do the impossible):

> Oh dear, Skylab is falling
> Oh dear, it's so appalling
> Oh dear, Saint Peter is calling
> I sure hope it won't fall on me.
> Falling from a great height
> Ooops—Chicken Little was right.
>
> The chances are likely it will not fall on us
> It's probable Skylab will not fall upon us
> Nothing's for sure—it's the will of the gods
> Even Jimmy the Greek won't give odds.
>
> I'm praying that it will not land where it shouldn't
> While they keep on saying that it could but it wouldn't
> With Congress dispersing—they're all heading home
> Out of fear that it might hit the Capitol dome.
> So what—it'll all be the same, Carter will still get the
>   blame.
>
> Will it hit Altoona? Don't make the inference
> That if it lands on Cleveland, we'll not know the differ-
>   ence.
> If it hits the Dakotas, Bismarck or Pierre,
> They could use the excitement up there.
>
> So Skylab is falling, we're in a fine fettle,
> How did we inherit these fish in a kettle.
> They make no umbrellas for hot molten metal,
> I sure hope it won't fall on me.

Since the prodigal Skylab was expected to return to Earth soon, time was a-wastin'. Homecoming preparations are always exciting, and every town within fifty degrees north and fifty degrees south of the equator vied for the honor of being the crash site. Skylab fever gripped the nation and various announcements began to appear: "Remember, pieces of the space craft will become the sole property of the survivors. In the event that (heaven forbid) Skylab crashes into the ocean, the offer is withdrawn. It's wise to order your hardhats and window shields now while the supply lasts. Send now for your official entry blank in the Skylab Sweepstakes. Those guessing the exact time and location of the crash will receive an all-expense-paid weekend at the fabulous San Andreas Motor Inn and Fault in sunny California. All three networks will be standing by to provide on-the-spot coverage of the Skylab plopdown. If it occurs in prime time, however, the broadcast will be delayed unless the crash takes place in either Times Square or the Loop in Chicago."

But, alas, it was not to be. The promise that Skylab held now lies on the floor of the Indian Ocean, belonging to history along with other Great Fizzles—Comet Kohoutek, "Supertrain," and "Don't Be Fuelish" stickers. Skylab must be considered a truly great fizzle because it held us in suspense for nearly a year. And that's something in this age of the six-second attention span.

Sure, we would have liked to see the raining debris sending people scurrying in all directions (in some other city than our own, of course), but as Socrates once said, "You can't have your hemlock and drink it too."

Good-by, Skylab. You were a nice diversion. Now it's back to gasoline, back to Iran, back to inflation. And thank you, NASA; you gave us quite a turn. We needed that.

While scientists may dazzle the world with their awesome accomplishments of massive proportions, I am more impressed with the little things such as the announcement by a major manufacturer that it was coming out with a $10 light bulb that would last five years. That is fine, but what we really need is a $10 bill that lasts five days. A five-year bulb could practically eliminate the thrill of replacing light bulbs on the ceiling. There's nothing like standing up on a chair and removing the globe, only to get a faceful of dead mosquitos.

It all started with Edison, who saw the need for inventing the electric light when the candle in his refrigerator kept going out. Scientists are now working on a refrigerator bulb that turns off when you open the door. It's for food that's afraid of the dark. Well, if they can make a light bulb that lasts five years, they could put a show on NBC that'll do the same thing. Good old Yankee ingenuity, that's what that five-year bulb is. Incidentally, Edison's first incandescent bulb is still burning, which I think sets a terrible example of wasting energy. Thank you, good night, and don't forget to turn out the lights. Unless, of course, you're a big investor in your local light and power company.

18. Depressions—7, Cures—0

During the Bicentennial, we celebrated the wondrous fact that this country was, at last, one hundred and sixty-seven years old—celsius.

HOW TO COUNT OUR PROBLEMS AND MEASURE OUR FAILURES—IN METRIC

I know that metric is inevitable. I realize that one day my little wide-eyed grandchildren are going to snuggle up to me and say, "Grandpa, tell us about the quart" as we look at my collection of antique glass containers.

"Well, Mary Sue, a long long time ago, me and your grandmaw, we had it rough. We had to buy things by the yard and the foot and the inch and the gallon. Yessiree, back in the old days we didn't know a liter from a kilogram."

"Hee-hee—oh, grandpa, tell us some more about the pioneer days. . . ."

Yes, metric is coming, but I'll be all right. I'm trying to stay cheerful. Before outlining my fear of the metric system any further, let me explain that I am not one of those to whom metric is the last extreme right-wing conservative issue. I don't equate new weights and measures with the Panama Canal treaty or Alger Hiss.

Don't include me in the crowd that says, "Aha, I knew it! Once we started Social Security and then let all them pinkos into the State Department, the next thing we knew, they tried to take away our God-given pound!" No, I don't even believe in Big Brother.

The John Birch Society crowd aren't the only ones who think the adoption of this system is a silly waste of time. Joining them are the 77 percent of us who, according to various polls, are against it. Who are the other 23 percent? Well, I've met some of them and they are awfully good at mathematics. They also seem to be high school teachers who are very condescending as they puff on their pipes and give a look that seems to say, "You ignoramus, you really can't see the big picture, can you?"

The main argument of the metric proponents is that the large American firms doing business with foreign countries are working at a disadvantage without it. In other words, our prestige around the world goes into the septic tank unless the thermometer outside the bank gives the temperature in Celsius. So there you have the 23 percent who are school teachers bored with teaching the old system and the multinational corporations versus the rest of us.

If there are any others in that 23 percent, perhaps they are just plain housewives who do business with Switzerland. And all those midwestern shoe salesmen who sell tractor parts to Yugoslavia.

But we the Digital Majority shall be heard. If it means metric civil war, so be it. A yardstick divided against itself cannot stand. I know not what course others may take, but as for me, give me liberty or give me cubic centimeters. I regret that I have but one illegal gallon jug to hide from my country. The Metric Minority doesn't care that most of us are against it. All they want is their kilogram of flesh.

Since the arrival of the metric system to our shores is inevitable, there's no sense brooding about it. So let's be positive and think of all the good that will come about. Metric will enable us to deal with the many problems that face this nation. Job crisis? Thanks to metric, we will be able to measure unemployment lines in kilometers. Energy? We'll make real progress when we can measure the high-priced imported oil in liters. Racial tension? Metric will bring us all together, because most people of all races, creeds, colors, and national origin are uniformly indifferent to it.

So think positive. Sure, metric will continue to have its detractors, but once the system catches on and we're all converted, we'll realize how much fun a real waste of time can be.

Now that you are convinced of the virtues of this new system, we might as well learn some of the terms—time's a wastin', so let's go. The Let's Cram Metric Down Their Throats Association, Ltd., has come out with a handy conversion guide. We are told that a centimeter is the width of a paper clip. A millimeter is the thickness of a paper clip. This next one is rather exotic—the hectare. A hectare is 2½ acres. They don't tell you how many paper clips. Someday in a Western movie, a rancher will say, "You mosey down the trail about fourteen kilometers and you come to my spread—the prettiest five thousand hectares in all of Texas."

If you wish to preserve yet another endangered part of the American way of life, write today. Send one dollar ($1.00) in care of Save Our Children from Metric. I promise to put that money to work, after expenses, of course, to help get the kilometer out of the classroom and back into foreign films where it belongs.

PUT PRINCE ALBERT BACK IN THE CAN
AND LET THE PRINGLES OUT

Very few things depress me as much as Pringles. Talk about the deterioration of the quality of life in America today—Pringles are a shame. And shame on Proctor and Gamble for making them. They should've stuck with soap. I'm not alone in my depression. Psychiatrists are all too familiar with the complaint: "It's not my childhood, doctor. Nor my mother nor my marriage. It's Pringles."

A few years ago when Pringles canned potato chips hit the marketplace and kids all over America, including my own, took to them in a big way, I realized how lucky I was as a child. When we were kids, potato chips didn't come packed in an airtight tennis ball can. When we were kids, when America was innocent, potato chips were the way they were meant to be—born free! Bouncing around in total freedom in a bag.

It's the uniform appearance of these little Formicalike potato poker chips that bothers me. Bringing them into the home, exposing our children to such a mundane product, can only have a dulling effect on their lives. Buy a Pringle in Maine, and then go to Oregon and buy another Pringle; if you hold them up together, you'll find that they are exactly the same. I've figured it all out. There is only *one* Pringle in the world. Only one—they keep it in a vault in the factory. The mother Pringle. All the others are clones.

The Pringle is technology run amok. Where Proctor and Gamble took innocent potatoes, dehydrated them, squeezed the moisture from their little bodies, and locked them up inside Alcoa aluminum and heavy cardboard tennis ball cans. Mark my word, the day will come when Dupont will take tennis balls and, you guessed it, put them inside of cellophane potato chip bags.

I was talking about this on television several years ago and mistakenly said that Pringles were made by Kraft. I soon received a letter from the public relations division of Kraft Foods, Inc. It said: "Sir: Be advised that our company, Kraft Foods, Inc. does not make Pringles. Pringles are made by Proctor and Gamble. However, we at Kraft Foods, Inc. make a dandy dip that goes nicely with them."

I replied: "Dear Kraft Foods, Inc. I stand corrected. I did not know that Pringles were made by Proctor and Gamble. But come to think of it, since they also make Ivory soap, this explains not only the Pringle taste, but also the fact that the little critters float."

The quality of life in the home can be uplifted by talking about Dr. Arno Penzias around your kids. Perhaps you've forgotten who Dr. Arno Penzias is. He is a Nobel Prize winner, for physics.

Are there Arno Penzias posters adorning any twelve-year-old's bedroom walls? Why not? How about any other American Nobel Prize winners? What about Hamilton Smith? (Medicine—I know, you forgot.) Herbert Simon? Isaac Bashevis Singer? Let's give these eggheads the recognition they deserve and make their names household words, right up there with Elvis, Bo Derek, Robert Redford, and Arthur Burns. (Arthur Burns fascinates me. I like to think that everyone remembers where they were on Pearl Harbor Day, what they were doing the day Kennedy was shot, and where they were when Arthur Burns left the Federal Reserve.)

Let's make a liar out of Alexander Solzhenitsyn, who said Americans are superficial and lacking in values. I want to see an America where any eighth-grader will fight for an Arno Penzias bubble-gum card—a nation where no decent self-respecting father would hesitate to buy two extra quarter pounders with cheese so that his kids can drink from a cup proudly bearing a picture of Herbert Simon (economics). And one day we can hope to see a winner of the Nobel Prize on our twenty-one-inch screens, proclaiming, "Before I head for the lab every morning, I make sure I'm fortified with a fiber cereal."

One way to bring this all about is for the whole family to sing the Arno Penzias Fight Song, to the tune of "Mister Touchdown, U.S.A.":

They always call him Mister Physics,
They always call him Mister "P,"
He's the champion in the lab,
And a Nobel Prize winner is he.
Hip, hip, hurray for Arno Penzias,
The king of the physicists by far;
He's a thermodynamic John Travolta
And a quantum theory superstar.

Come on, make way for Isaac Singer,
Hey, there's a writer that's for sure.
We always knew that he would win
The prize for literature.
Come, put his name on every sneaker.
For Singer tee shirts there must be a need,
And his name will be known on every college campus
If only the students could read.

MID-LIFE IS NOT AN INSURANCE COMPANY

It has been only a couple of years since writers of books and magazines discovered middle-aged people and their mid-life crises. That term "mid-life" bothers me. It implies that you're ready for the Boy Scout to help you cross the street. Apparently we have never been interesting enough to warrant books and magazine articles until we reached middle age. When we graduated from high school in the late forties or early fifties, nobody paid us any attention. We missed World War II, and when Korea is mentioned these days, it's only in reference to bribes.

We knew nothing of the stuff of youthful glory—panty raids, crowding into phone booths, burning draft cards, hiding in Canada, dropping acid, and snorting coke. In school, we behaved. When drafted, we went. We toed the mark, obeyed, conformed—and were ignored. We were dull.

Suddenly we became fascinating. We were discovered in the late seventies when anxiety over Vietnam and Watergate changed to anxiety over matters of a more personal nature. The Tet offensive, napalm, Ho Chi Minh, Haldeman, Dean, and the tapes were traded in for taxes, depression, inflation, and divorce—which meant that it was our turn in the limelight.

Some of us in this dangerous, difficult mid-life time of turmoil attempted to cope by embracing more than one culture. To maintain our own identities and still be aware of the hip contemporary scene is not easy for those of us who struggle daily to keep from falling behind in today's frenzied pace. Not easy for those of us who think Fleetwood Mac is a Cadillac dealer. Not easy for those of us who think Arnold Schwartzenegger was the prime minister who succeeded the Kaiser. Not easy for those of us who think Beverly Sills is the name of a California window frame company. Not easy for those of us who think that Richard Dreyfuss was the guy on Devil's Island. Not easy for those of us who think that Sha Na Na once ruled Iran. And not easy for all of us who think that Macho was an unknown Marx brother.

Sure, I've smoked marijuana—many of us going through midlife crisis have. My problem is that I have to be reminded to pass it around. I tried cocaine once, and believe me, never again. It was a disaster. It kept falling out of my nose, landing all over my tie. People asked me about it. They said clever things like, "Say, I believe you've got white powder all over your tie. What is that?"

I'd say, "Oh, that? Tooth powder."

They'd say, "You brush your teeth with your tie on?"

I'd say, "Yeah—what about it?"

They'd say, "Why?"

I'd say, "I'm a Virgo—we're very, very neat."

Then I'd start sneezing like crazy until everyone left me alone—and I blew all the powder off my tie.

HERE'SYOURCHANGETHANKYOUAND
HAVEANICEDAY

Recently, a friend's child was flying across the country alone, to be met by his father at the airport. You can imagine my friend's anxiety when the plane was nearly three hours late. During the agonizing moments of uncertainty as to the plane's whereabouts, he called the airline repeatedly for information. At each attempt, the clerk ended the conversation by saying, "We don't know where the plane is, thank you for calling American, and have a nice day."

This essay is not a criticism of airlines, this is an all-out attack on "have a nice day." How many times during your day do people command you to have a nice one? When the cashier in the lunch counter stares into the cash register and mumbles, "Have a nice day," did you ever wonder if she was wishing the nice day to you or to the money in the drawer? When the bank official, having turned down your request for a loan, peers over his glasses and murmurs, "Have a nice day," how nice will it be without the money?

Hasn't this gratuitous, programmed little speech of phony well-wishing gone far enough? If I want to have a nice day, I'll have a nice day, but I want the right to choose and not have it forced on me by uncaring strangers.

I believe we can pinpoint the origin of the mass use of this ersatz good cheer to, of all things, the Vietnam War. Hippies, at least the less militant ones, said it to the police as they were being dragged into the paddy wagons. Peaceniks said it as they put flowers into police gun barrels. Our national morale was so rotten in the sixties that not only did it seem important to start wishing each other a nice day, but it also gave rise to the mandatory insipid "happy talk" on local news shows. But in these comparatively peaceful times, both should be abolished in the name of national honesty— and sanity.

Several variations on "have a nice day" can be heard on the ABC show with the equally cheerful title "Good Morning, America." Host David Hartman, who one day is surely to be sent to the Home for the Chronically Pleasant, ends each show with not so much a cliche, but a challenge: "Make it a good day." Good for David; that's the old Puritan ethic—you've got to go out and work for it. That is much more uplifting than Rona Barrett's old sign-off, "Keep thinkin' the good thoughts." So with David and Rona, "Good Morning, America" started us off each day with a blend of Emerson and Charlie Brown.

I think, if I had a morning show, I'd close each day by revealing my true feelings: "Have a nice day—and if you don't, I'll never speak to you again."

FILTHY PHONE CALLS THAT SELL

Our lives are controlled by research. Opinion gathering is an enormous industry whose basic method is to ask us what we like, run it through a computer, and proceed to tell us what we want.

Somewhere, someone took a survey and concluded that what people want are junk phone calls. Apparently millions of people, never before polled, have been sitting around, all thinking the same thought: "Boy, what I wouldn't give to be interrupted by an annoying commercial on the telephone right now." It follows that some market researcher said, "Our exhaustive studies show that the vast majority of the public welcomes the idea of advertising by phone. Our studies also show that most people enjoy eating raw liver and having root canal work done."

If junk phone calls are an idea whose time has come, we may also conclude that the same applies to obscene phone calls. Which ultimately will bring on the dawn of the combination junk obscene call—a sales pitch spiced with dirty words and heavy breathing.

WHAT'S RONG WITH THIS SENTENCE?

Going to a stand-up cocktail party? Ready to waste two hours clutching a wet napkin wrapped around a glass? How's your conversation going to be? Witty? Inspired? Or do you already have the fear that people are going to stare at your left ear as you regale them with your profundity that *Rocky* was a good movie?

Well, fear no more, because here is my secret of how to hold their attention! Like a good pitcher, the T.A.C. (Terribly Amusing Conversationalist) should make use of the change of pace. The trick is to give that old predictable statement a surprise ending. Someone walks up to you and opens with the universal greeting: "How are you?" No reply of "Fine" for you; you say, "My wallet was stolen yesterday and as far as I'm concerned, they can keep the irreplaceable sentimental pictures and driver's license, but what I really want to get back is the money." The person to whom you're speaking might think, "What a heartless grubber." In which case you wouldn't want to continue conversing with him anyway. Or else he, being as bored with the usual cocktail chitchat as you, will counter with, "That's true, but pickpockets always seem to know where people carry their sentimental pictures."

Some other variations on a theme are the following: "You know, Jim Nabors sings just the way he talks."

"A martini please—and don't spare the vermouth."

"My boy, I didn't go to college. Having more advantages than you, I'm lucky."

"If you take your eye off the ball and bend that left arm a bit, you'll play a better game of golf."

"The thing about Beethoven is, he was greatly appreciated in his own time."

"I have quite a vast knowledge of art, but I never quite know what I like."

"Arizona may be hotter, but it has less humidity. And it's just as miserable in the summer as back east."

"What a vacation. Now that it's over, I've got to stay off my diet."

"Novocain—now that's entertainment!"

I must warn you that there is a certain risk involved in using these on strangers. Your sanity could become suspect, resulting in your being thrown out. So if you panic and wish to become one of the crowd again, simply revert back to such safe and sane stand-bys as:

"How about those Rams yesterday?"

"A lot of people just don't know how to drive in this kind of weather."

"After Labor Day we've got the whole beach to ourselves."

"Kids sure know more today than we did at that age."

"I get about 16 on the highway, 14 in town."

"I'm just afraid some nut is going to take a shot at him."

"I just don't eat desserts, that's all."

"*Rocky* sure was a good movie."

The rest is up to you. Almost anything will do as long as it's stale, trite, and utterly predictable.

WRITE OR WIRE COLLECT OR CALL MY PERSONAL TOLL-FREE NUMBER

I don't know when it all started to go wrong between Grace Kelly and me. It was the real thing, all right—in fact I almost went to jail for her. It was 1953 and I was in the Marine Corps waiting at the Navy embarkation station on Treasure Island in San Francisco Bay to be shipped out. As my outfit received its orders and was assigned a troop ship, I was ashore in a movie theatre watching *To Catch a Thief* for the seventh time. I risked the brig for the woman who had been the object of my love ever since St. Paul's Elementary School.

We learned from the priests and nuns and the publicity how perfect Grace was. She was on the same pedestal in our young minds as the Virgin Mary. "That's the kind of girl you should want, boys," the priests would say, and from then on, whenever I heard the term "sanctifying grace," I assumed they were referring to the beautiful, talented, and wealthy blonde from that good Catholic family of Philadelphia.

In my travels, I have met a lot of guys who, like me, have been walking around staring blankly into space, not quite recovered from that initial shock of the announcement so many years ago that Grace would marry that dandy Prince Rainier of Monaco. Some don't admit too readily to be still carrying the torch, but when I convince them that I, too, know what it's been like, they finally break down and let loose.

It usually goes like this as they blurt out: "Yes, yes, yes. I admit it. It's been nearly thirty years and I still search the TV listings hoping to find *Country Girl*, *High Society*, or even *High Noon*! My wife knows, but we never talk about it. Grace Kelly was perfection itself, too good for me, sure, and of course it's too much to hope that she'll leave her husband and run away with me." Sometimes, the sobbing becomes so pathetic, I must turn away.

We are out there. A silent fan club, if you will. Being too old for such foolishness, we have no meetings, no posters, and none of the tacky worship symbols. Grace Kelly just stands above all the other objects of male idolatry, before her time or since. We guard the pedestal she stands upon, not really wanting her to step down from it. What I'm saying is, Charlie's Angels couldn't shine Grace's tiara.

In spite of these feelings, I did a strange thing when Princess Caroline, Grace's daughter, was married. You may recall that the wedding was an extravagant affair, attended by international jet set celebs and given wide press coverage. I poked fun at these nuptials. It's my stock in trade to do so, but perhaps what I did, considering my deep relationship with the bride's mother, would be found interesting to a shrink.

It was an immature thing to do, but not having received an invitation to the wedding, I printed the following announcement in my newspaper column:

> So your invitation to Princess Caroline's wedding in Monaco never came? Well, don't panic. Send now for the Do-It-Yourself At-Home Monaco Wedding Kit! Be the first in your neighborhood to be an idle, disgustingly rich gadabout without leaving the house. The kit contains two Monaco travel posters, Cheese Doodles, frozen dip, two splits of Blue Nun, and a 45 RPM of "Oh, Promise Me" sung by Jim Nabors. As an added bonus, you get life-sized statues of the princess and her groom, Phillipe Junot, in heavy cardboard with two round holes to insert the heads of you and your friends. Don't wait! The Monaco Wedding Kit is our greatest home entertainment offer since our wildly popular Princess Margaret Divorce Game.

If you are one of Those Who Can't Forget Her, let us raise our glasses, think of Grace in the picnic scene in *To Catch A Thief*, and sing our song once again:

> Oh, she never calls, she never writes, and she never
>   thinks of me,
> But her picture has been hanging on my wall for a
>   quarter century.

AND THAT REMINDS ME . . .

They're cranking up Camp David again. So, get ready for more hugging.

   Try and picture this cartoon in a recent issue of *The New Yorker.* We see a family gathered in the kitchen. The two young children, a boy and a girl, are at the kitchen table neatly doing their homework, smiling. Mom is diligently cooking while smiling. Dad is busy fixing a broken appliance, wearing a beatific smile. And an elderly grandpa walks into the room smiling as the rest of the family gives him a loving and cheerful greeting. The caption under the cartoon says: "This is a simulated picture." The implication, of course, is that the 1980 family kitchen is rarely, if ever, that placid, rosy, and perfect. Similarly, scenes and pictures giving as fake an impression as this cartoon family can be found in the pages of our daily newspapers, as well as on the six o'clock news. I'm thinking about that fake picture during the Camp David summit meeting of Anwar Sadat hugging Menachem Begin, then Jimmy Carter hugging Menachem Begin, then Anwar Sadat hugging Jimmy Carter, then Jimmy Carter hugging Menachem Begin again. Then they all left Camp David, drove over to the Capitol building, and everybody hugged Tip O'Neill. What was the meaning of this hug-a-thon? I honestly forgot. And they interrupted Sunday night TV to act out this simulated picture. They should all sign another agreement which says: Don't hug me unless you love me.

When she gave her hand to someone else, that she loved
   me not was plain,
And since that day I have not known a moment without
   out pain.
But I will wait for you, Grace Kelly, though you don't
   know that I exist.
And with your prince there in your palace, you'll never
   know what you have missed.

When I was a lad back in '53, my dreams were all of
   Grace and me.

And of the day I'd pack up and go, when she'd order
me to Monaco.
Perhaps some day she'll come to know the truth, and
then at last
She'll realize that those years with him were all a
wasted past.

My hope through all these years has been that she'd
face reality
And gladly give her kingdom up for just one hour with
me.
We'd settle down in a little place. She'd be known as
the former Princess Grace.
She'd forget that place called Monaco—in our trailer
park near Buffalo.

I will wait for you, Grace Kelly, through this prolonged
anxiety.
When will you ever make your mind up?
Is it Rainier or is it—me?

19. These Are All Lies, Smear Tactics, Innuendo, A Fishing Expedition—And I'll Never Do It Again!

Sock it to me?   —RICHARD NIXON, 1968

When it comes to capturing the mood of America, presidential
candidates are right up there with the other great mood-cap-
turers—MacDonald's, Adidas, and the American Broadcasting

Company. They know what Americans want—cheeseburgers, sneakers, and the number-one show for a long time, "Three's Company."

And that's why, every four years, they dust off the greatest crowd pleaser of all—blaming Washington. Blaming Washington is the new snake oil. It'll give you as much pleasure as cheeseburgers, sneakers, and Suzanne Somers jumpin' up and down. When you combine blamin' Washington with a little Sunday mornin' preachin'—my friends, that'll go down smoother than a slug o' corn likker on a hot summer's evenin'.

Now, ya gotta know the rules. Ya cain't blame Washington while yer sittin' right in it, can ya? Nope. That's why ya gotta skeedaddle right outta there and go out into the heartland and tell 'em how Washington's an island. It worked in '76 and it'll work again. And ya gotta make 'em forget that the island is inhabited by the very bureaucracy chosen by the very people they put there. And don't let 'em remember that all those bad ole congressmen come from their own hometowns. Tell the folks that only you can lead them into the sunshine of pride and patriotism that comes only with blamin' Washington.

Jimmy Carter's highly successful run for the presidency in 1976 succeeded, I believe, because it was an anti-Washington campaign. It was wise and politically astute for him to run such a campaign, given the attitude of the public toward the city since Watergate. Carter's campaign theme seemed to be, "Washington is rotten to the core, and I want to go there." Ironically, by the time he was halfway through with his first term, it became apparent that he was the guy he had been warning us about.

As I travel around the United States, I occasionally tell someone that I'm from Washington, and the reaction is, "Well, you don't know what's going on in the rest of the country." Or I hear how fed up everyone is with the place. That expression, "fed up," is the quickie, catch-all rallying cry of many people outside of the nation's capital, signifying that everything from high prices to the heartbreak of psoriasis can easily be blamed on this place on the map called Washington, or on that longer, single-word description, "themessinwashington."

It seems that everything blessed, pure, and beautiful is found in Kansas, or Georgia, or Iowa, or anywhere but the source of everything evil and nasty, Washington. I wonder what people in all those other places would do without this oversimplified scapegoat. But if there is horrid corruption, bungling chicanery, and stupidity (and there is), where did all those boobs come from? They came from Kansas, Georgia, and Iowa, that's where. And the reason everything is so pure in the rest of the country is because you sent all of your scoundrels to Washington. They're not from here; they're from *there*. *You* sent them here to give us a bad reputation, and then you won't even let us have voting rights in Congress.

It became particularly traumatic for us permanent Washingtonians in 1977, during the time of the Bert Lance affair. As a member of the Washington media, I had to claim full responsibility for anything Bert Lance might have done that was not totally squeaky clean and saintly. Lance blamed the Washington media for his troubles, and he was correct. You see, before he made any financial decisions, Bert Lance would first call me for advice. I would always say, "Bert, you're the Georgia banker and I'm just a Washington media person. So my advice is to do whatever you've always done."

Look at every check Bert Lance ever wrote, and it'll be in my handwriting. Same with Carter's speeches. What drove me to it? Blind ambition.

One particular incident demonstrates how the Carter White House might have avoided embarrassment had they been a little more experienced with life as it is in Washington. The White House attempted to take off the air a TV commercial for the *Washington Star* newspaper, which showed a Doonesbury cartoon of the White House combined with an imitation of President Carter's voice. By trying to stop the commercial, the White House fell into an old trap. By showing anger, they drew more attention to the commercial than the commercial otherwise would have drawn.

It has been my experience that if a public figure happens to be present when jokes are being told at his expense, he reacts in one of the following ways: a) He may swallow hard, clench his teeth, and force the corners of his mouth as far apart as possible, holding the counterfeit grin for at least ten seconds. It's painful, but chances are he will be dubbed "a good sport"—if not a grinning fool. b) He may just sit there without a trace of expression on his face as the jokes seem to ricochet off him, all the time wishing he were home doing something fun like reading his hate mail. c) He may stand up red-faced in front of everyone and declare, "I am offended, and I demand that you cease." That was the reaction the White House chose and it's the worst one. If they had only used reaction "a" or "b" one of the networks would not have done what it did. It ran the commercial as a news story free of charge, to be seen by the whole country.

Those of us who live here cry and bleed, burn our toast, and get letters from collection agencies just like other mortals. All has not been Camelot here. The British burned the town in the War of 1812, and since then we have seen some mean times during which we again fit the description of a "war-torn capital."

Washington became a city of darkness and gloom when President Carter, with one stroke of his pen, eliminated the free parking spaces for thousands of government workers. I don't know if people around the rest of the country realize what it means to a government worker when he loses his free parking space, but here in Washington to be stripped of this coveted possession means public disgrace, a defrocking if you will, as thousands of stenciled names on those spaces are unceremoniously painted over as if they never existed.

Once these civil servants had it all. Now, as the list of the doomed was being drawn up, some knew they would be spared—congressmen, for example. But in many Washington homes they waited, hoping and praying that their names would not be on the list, so nobody would ever say to their children, "I can't play with you because your father lost his space."

Two words that show up in the news with alarming frequency are "bribery" and "conspiracy." For some time now, it has seemed that a day without bribery and conspiracy is like a day without politics.

I started to be aware of the frequency of the B&C charge on a day several years ago when one former congressman, one current congressman, and one Washington, D.C., local official, all on the same day, were indicted for bribery and conspiracy. Also on that day, a fourth politician was arraigned and charged with soliciting

an undercover policeman for sex. In his case, he was the only one
of the four showing any imagination.

It's getting to the point where newspapers will have to run a
permanent department along with the weather, horoscope, and the
ball scores and call it "Your Daily Bribery & Conspiracy Update."
Newspapers are always looking for ways to liven up their pages,
and the B&C of the day would rival "Blondie and Dagwood" for
sheer light-hearted fun. As Jimmy the Greek gives the morning
line on who might be the next politician to get nailed on a B&C,
betting in the office pool could take up the slack after the football
season.

It becomes increasingly difficult to keep track of the number of
people charged with good old B&C. I hope the day never comes
when a newspaper runs a banner headline declaring, "Congressman Frebish put in an inspiring, unselfish day today," as if it
were surprising news.

This is not to agree with Mark Twain's comment about Congress being a notorious criminal class. That is a bit harsh. We must
assume they are all innocent—until they learn the ropes.

The bribery and conspiracy charge is becoming so boring that
they'll soon start booking office holders on suspicion of virtue.

Senator Herman Talmadge, on the other hand, was just plain
flat-out guilty. Not of the things he was charged with, but for giving us the poorest excuse for a scandal in the history of political
hijinks. I can honestly say that I heard absolutely no one in Washington discuss the case. If there were any Talmadge jokes, I didn't
hear them. Not one person asked me what I thought of Talmadge.
If anyone had, my answer would have been, "I don't think of Talmadge, especially while I'm driving, because I might plow into
something."

Look at the charges: that he converted campaign contributions
to his personal use. Now how original was that? They ought to
throw the book at him for blatant lack of imagination. Where's
Fanne Foxx? Elizabeth Ray? Moonlight swims in the Tidal Basin?
All we had was an ex-wife who says she got her money from an
overcoat. Yippee. And he calls himself a public servant. As if Talmadge weren't boring enough, his hearings were conducted by
that magnetic firebrand of the senate, Adlai Stevenson III, who's
been known to make "Scoop" Jackson look like the

Marx Brothers. Senator Talmadge has been around long enough to
know that the old financial mismanagement trap won't get you
those big headlines, and when applied to a politician, it just isn't
news any more.

One story typical of the inner workings of Washington unfolded
during a time when Congress had to pass judgment on one of its
own. When the House of Representatives voted *not* to expel Congressman Charles Diggs of Michigan, even though he was found
guilty of 29 counts of taking salary kickbacks, I figured it was because Diggs got in right under the wire, since the cut-off point is
30 counts. As a member of the House, Diggs voted on behalf of
himself (surprise), and I imagined his statement: "I wrestled with
this one, but finally I had to vote my conscience." Congressman
Diggs voted in favor of keeping his own job.

  Right after Diggs's unsurprising vote on his own behalf, Republican leader John Rhodes leaped to his feet. (Nobody in Congress ever just stands; they always leap to their feet.) He shouted,
"Point of order" an expression that is the closest thing in the
House to "bull feathers." Then Democratic leader Jim Wright of
Texas made an impassioned speech, which is the only kind he ever
makes. When Wright hails a cab he does it with passion. He said
the only time House members were expelled was back in 1861 for
joining the Confederate Congress. All of this should prompt Hollywood to redo the old Jimmy Stewart movie of the thirties and
call it *Mr. Diggs Stays in Washington.*

In case you're thinking that nothing goes on in Washington but
graft and corruption, let me relate to you a heart-warming story of
a longtime attempt by a lobbying organization to exert what I
thought to be blatant influence upon the entire United States Senate, only to be rebuffed by all 100 members of that august body.
Are we talking about cigar-chewing defense contractors wining
and dining our lawmakers? No. Are we talking about Korean lobbyists sneaking envelopes stuffed with hundred-dollar bills under
the table? No, scandal fans. Vicuña coats, champagne, free trips to
exotic places, what you call your *femmes fatales?* None of these.
We're talking about snuff.

  I had always known that the Senate had an age-old tradititon of keeping a fresh supply of snuff on hand at all times, placing it in containers at each of the two entrances to the Senate chamber. I suppose that at one time this was a practical convenience, but it could hardly be so in this age of the jogging Senator Proxmire and two (count 'em) Senate gymnasiums.

Being curious about the mechanics of the senatorial snuff supply, I wanted to interview, on television, the person who actually filled the containers; certainly the viewers would like to know that there is such a person in the government and would want to hear about his unusual occupation. Where is the bulk of the snuff kept? How much is consumed over a given period of time? Where does it come from? Do the taxpayers pay for it? The public has a right to know, and besides, "Sixty Minutes" can't do it all.

I had hardly begun my venture into investigative reporting when I hit the stone wall. A correct and precise sergeant-at-arms of the Senate reminded me that absolutely no pictures can ever be taken inside the Senate chamber. He also said he didn't know who filled the snuff boxes, nor did he know where the bulk of the snuff was stored. I asked him if he could get this information for me, and he referred me to the maintenance department of the Capitol Building. The maintenance department of the Capitol is more knowledgeable of the government process than the sergeant-at-arms; they knew immediately that the master container of snuff is kept in the men's room. It was under the jurisdiction of one of the custodians, a Mr. Brown, known to all in the department as "Brownie." Obviously, Brownie was my man and I would put him on television.

No way. I was thwarted in my many attempts to contact Brownie through phone calls, messages, and personal visits. I then tried another angle. I discovered that although the level of the snuff in the boxes kept going down, no senator used it. Obviously there was a phantom snuff sniffer. The name of this person was surreptitiously given to me by a friend who is a Capitol Hill employee. All I can reveal is that he has access to the Senate chamber.

With a zeal that would make Woodward and Bernstein envious, I asked the snuff user the identity of the supplier of the snuff to the Capitol, how often delivery was made, and in what amount. In a barely audible whisper over the phone (from a phone booth, natu-

rally) the sniffer said, "The snuff is sent from the Smokeless Tobacco Institute in Peekskill, New York." At last, the break I was
waiting for.

ME: Good afternoon. This is Mark Russell in Washington. I'd like
   some information about the snuff that I understand your organization sends to the Capitol Building here from time to
   time.
SMOKELESS TOBACCO SPOKESMAN: Yes?
ME: I guess the person I'm looking for would be your public infor-
   mation officer.
S. T. S.: Well, uh, I guess that would be me.
ME: Oh, fine. Tell me, how long has the Smokeless Tobacco Insti-
   tute been shipping snuff to the U.S. Senate, anyway?
S. T. S.: Well, it's an old tradition dating back about a hundred and
   fifty years when many senators used snuff.
ME: I see—and how often do you send it?
S. T. S. (rather guardedly): Uh, well, uh, no specific timetable.
ME (bearing down): Well, would it be once a week or once a
   month, or what?
S. T. S.: Maybe, uh, once a month. Sometimes, maybe, uh, once a
   month.
ME: Once a month. I see. And tell me, exactly what volume of
   snuff goes out in these monthly shipments?
S. T. S.: One can.
ME: One can. But how big is the can? Are we talking about a fifty-
   gallon drum or something smaller?
S. T. S.(growing slightly suspicious): We send one four-ounce can.
ME (slightly patronizing): Forgive me, not being in the business, I
   don't know, but exactly how big is a four-ounce container?
S. T. S (very suspicious): It would be a can a little less than half the
   size of a normal soup can.
ME (informed): Ah, I see—and you've been sending a can of snuff,
   a little less than half the size of a normal soup can, to the Senate in Washington about once a month for a hundred and fifty
   years.
S. T. S. (feigning patience): That is correct.
ME (preparing to fire the salvo): Do you charge the Senate for the
   snuff?

S. T. S. (dropping guard, rapidly losing patience): Of course not. This is a courtesy we simply extend as a goodwill gesture that has been a part of American history.

ME (unimpressed, launching salvo): Don't you think that by not charging for the snuff, the Smokeless Tobacco Institute is attempting to apply undue influence upon United States Senators?

S. T. S. (after a long silence): What—did—you—say?

ME: I said, don't you think that by not charging . . .

S. T. S.: I heard you. Absolutely not. Did you say you were calling from Washington? Who are you—are you in the media? You're with the media, aren't you? This conversation is finished.

CLICK.

So much for hardball journalism. As I mentioned, this is a heartwarming story because no senator takes advantage of this blatant dumping of four ounces of snuff a month. Which shows that the post-Watergate morality is casting an encouraging spell over our lawmakers. The only one actually partaking of the favors is my source, the phantom snuff sniffer. As I said, his identity will not be revealed here. We'll just call him "Deep Nose."

20. Anatomy of a Banquet

I confess ignorance about dozens of subjects (okay, thousands), but there is one topic on which I must claim to be an unqualified expert. That subject is banquets. Did I say "unqualified expert"? Make that "infallible." If banquets were faith and dogma, I would be Pope. If they were home runs, I would be Hank Aaron. Most meals I have had in the past twenty years were eaten at banquets, since most of the shows I have done outside of Washington were done at banquets. I have spent my adult life at the Head Table, but

not without paying the penalty. All those tablecloths have given
me lint lung.

It has reached the point where during the busy banquet season
in the spring or fall, even if I am in a restaurant alone, I'll automatically stand to salute the flag, and won't order until the maitre 'd
gives the benediction. I have spoken everywhere, from the Waldorf to ghetto nursing homes, from embassy garden parties to a big
event in New Jersey that required white tie—and black shirts.

Under our system, the more banquets you attend, the better you
are doing, the more important you are in your line of work. For
example, if you are a mechanic working for a car dealer, perhaps
your boss, the Oldsmobile King, will have the annual Christmas
party for the whole gang—sales, parts, accounting, and the service
department, which includes you (and often is *only* you). So for
this once-a-year bash at the Holiday Inn the purchase of a tuxedo
isn't necessary.

But if you graduate from your shop coat to a white-collar sales
job up in the show room, you'll be going to more banquets. Soon
you'll be dining with your car sales colleagues—not only those
from the Oldsmobile King but others from the Chevrolet King and
the Dodge King. Yes, as a member of the Regional Automobile
Sales Association, you will be tasting your success with each nib-
ble of the best well-done steak the Ramada Inn has to offer. But remember, success has its price, paid to the dry cleaners (watch that
steak sauce), and since your wife naturally will be accompanying
you, to the hairdresser, the baby sitter, and the better-dress department of your local department store.

This is only the beginning for you. More steaks, baked potatoes
gift-wrapped in aluminum foil, and hearts of lettuce crowned with
diet mayonnaise await you at the State Automobile Sales Association. There's no stopping now—soon the chicken at the National
Automobile Sales Association Banquet will beckon. By now
you're hooked. You open your own place and at last *you* are the
Oldsmobile King. You now have a live-in maid, you own two tux-
edos, and your wife has a dozen wigs. You've just been elected
president of your local Automobile Dealers Association, which automatically shoots you into the Rotary, Kiwanis, Chamber of
Commerce, United Givers Fund, and the Symphony Board, even
though your favorite recording is by Hank Snow. You attend the

banquets of each of these groups and they all fall in October. The month is topped by the Annual Closing Banquet of the National Association of Automobile Dealers convening in Houston. This is the Big Time and you are at the head table. The chocolate mousse, having been set free from a three-day incarceration in the freezer, sits half-eaten before 1,200 guests. The speeches begin. Merciless salvos are hurled against Ralph Nader, auto emission standards, and the foreign menace, but you hear none of them, because you are asleep. It's been a long month.

If you are that member of the National Association of Automobile Dealers and attend all those banquets, I can still top you because I've not only spoken at your banquet, but also at those of the national associations of doctors, lawyers, manufacturers, teachers, peanut growers, gas producers (the banquet chefs notwithstanding), oil producers, scrap iron dealers, TV weatherpersons, and many more, including an association of people who work for their fathers called Sons of Bosses (SOBs).

When you are an expert on anything, you recognize the opportunities for improving that thing. The fact is that most banquets are planned in a very haphazard and unskilled manner by those who are too occupied with their own businesses. Therefore, I have prepared Mark Russell's Guidelines for the Banquet That Everyone Will Remember Long After They Leave the Parking Lot. My guidelines (I wouldn't be a Washingtonian without passing on a few guidelines now, would I?) fall into categories, each constituting a segment of a banquet. The categories are: 1) Cocktails and Receptions. 2) The Head Table Tradition. 3) The Invocation. 4) Introduction of the Members of the Head Table. 5) The Food. 6) The Music. 7) Speeches and Entertainment.

1) COCKTAILS. If an organization has a banquet and there is a cash bar at the reception, we know we are dealing with a very cheap outfit. The tacky business of lining up for tickets for drinks is okay at Disneyland, but if the organization can't afford the booze, then it is not as successful as the speeches later on will indicate.

The cocktail party ranks way up there with the great institutions of American life—the saloon brawl, the January White Sale, and the Battle of Gettysburg—as hundreds of bodies are thrown together in forced confrontation. Yet there is an air of childlike innocence at these affairs, since everyone has a cute little plastic badge with his name on it pinned to his clothing just like on the first day of kindergarten.

The ID tag is a practical way to deal with an identity crisis since the wearer merely glances down at his chest and reads not only his name but his organization. This is the civilian version of "name, rank, and serial number." So if an IBM cocktail party is attacked by guerillas from Honeywell and prisoners are taken, under the Geneva Convention they may give only the information printed on the name tag: "IBM Mid-Year Meeting, Palmer House, Chicago, Hi, My Name's Ernie, What's Yours?"

2) THE HEAD TABLE TRADITION. The reason for a Head Table is that its occupants would suffer heart murmurs if placed anywhere else. The Head Table is always a few feet higher than the ordinary round tables for the groundlings, because the members of the Head Table consider themselves to be on a higher plane than the others. The members of the Head Table (MOTHT) always enter the hall after the others are seated, amid all the pageantry that can be dreamed up. Remember, not only are the MOTHT the ones to be honored at a banquet, they are also the ones who planned the thing in the first place.

In the sixties, the composer Cy Coleman wrote the song "Hey, Look Me Over" for his musical *Wildcat*, but he probably never imagined that the song would be forever played by every banquet orchestra as the honored guests marched into the hall to take their places at the Head Table. Before the song was written, "Pomp and Circumstance" was played, and if the truth be known, this martial air is missed.

The Head Table is a phenomenon whose origins probably can be tracked back to the Last Supper—the idea of sitting on only one side of a long narrow table. Except that on *that* night there were no other tables in the room. I suppose the only others besides the Head Table guests and the waiter at the Last Supper was Leonardo de Vinci on the opposite side of the room with his paints.

3) THE INVOCATION. The Supreme Court may have taken prayer out of the public schools, but petitioning the Deity is still flourishing at banquets. The invocation by a priest, minister, or rabbi—or all three, as at the National Conference of Christians

and Jews banquet—is the seal of divine approval of the activities of the particular group.

I can think of no better example of the way in which we stereotype our clergy than the token task assigned to them at banquets. Unless the dinner is religious in nature, a man of the cloth is rarely invited for any other reason than to give the invocation—the calling upon heaven to bless not only the hotel food (a miracle?), but also the nefarious occupations of the guests. You would think that in these enlightened times any self-respecting servant of God would be wise to the fact that he is being used when called upon to perform this duty, but apparently not.

Just once, I would like to see this happen: A priest gets a call: "Uh, Father, we the National Association of Heating and Plumbing Contractors are having our convention at the Hilton next Tuesday, and we would like you to give the invocation." And the priest answers, "No way! I want to give the main speech!"

Sometimes the one giving the invocation is a special friend of the organization. If this is the case, everyone is in for a treat, because the prayer before the meal is usually personalized to fit the occasion. The invocation is tailor-made to apply to the group's particular activity, in an often hilarious attempt to improve upon Holy Writ.

There is an enormous sports banquet held annually in Washington by a group known as the Touchdown Club. It's a stag affair attended by 2,000 lobbyists and politicians who, following a three-hour cocktail party, file in for the boozy dinner and the speeches given by famous athletes, cabinet members, and the president or vice president. But for me the highlight of the evening is the invocation, which is always delivered by the chaplain of the club, Father Tom Kane, an eloquent priest whose voice echoes over the reeling crowd, beseeching the Almighty to "make the steaks tender, the speeches brief, and guide us along the gridiron of life to our final goal, and the extra point of eternity in the paradise hall of fame." Similarly, the Brunswick Corporation has a bowling chaplain. At their wing-ding he asks a blessing "that we make nothing but strikes in life and avoid the gutterballs of sin."

The shortest, most touching prayer I've ever witnessed at a banquet was delivered not by a clergyman but by the former baseball star Ted Williams. It was back in the late sixties and he had been given some award. Williams made a short speech of thanks, then, his voice rising, said, "God Bless Spiro Agnew!"

4) INTRODUCTION OF MEMBERS OF THE HEAD TABLE. This is absolutely the most crucial moment of any banquet. The dreary exercise of calling out the names of the MOTHT as they stand at their places can make or break any banquet. The culprit here is the master of ceremonies, who is also one of the honored guests. After attending thousands of banquets, I have concluded that the master of ceremonies is chosen after he wins the association's contest for dullest speaker. He wouldn't be at the Head Table if he didn't have a certain talent, but speaking into a microphone is rarely it.

I once was at the Head Table at a convention of dentists, and as I was sitting next to the lectern I could see the master of ceremonies' notes. At the top of the page in big bold type was printed, "GOOD EVENING, LADIES AND GENTLEMEN." Great ad-libbers, those dentists!

My favorite part of the introductions is when the emcee introduces his wife. This is always a touching moment and can be very revealing as to how he really feels about her. When introducing the wives, emcees often lay it on a little thick with tokens of undying love and affection, as if the entire audience had doubts about this particular marriage. The Head Table of a banquet always seems to me to be a strange place to renew one's vows. Emcees always use cutesy introductions such as, "Now I'd like you to meet the little gal who puts up with my nonsense all year long, the mother of our four wonderful children, who still finds time to do her chores every day—I love her because she takes her Geritol—here she is—my lifesmate—my copilot on the not-so-calm seas of matrimony—my lovely wife Doreen." Doreen dutifully stands, direct from the beauty shop and with a clenched Pat Nixon smile; she is probably thinking, "If I had married that nice young mechanic, I'd be sitting down there with the others having a good time."

5) THE FOOD. The mediocre dinners served up by hotels may not be a bad thing, since the food itself is often the banquet's best entertainment. Many a hearty laugh can be shared over the chicken à la Goodyear, past-its-prime beef.

Art Buchwald, speaking at a luncheon at the Shoreham several years ago, called attention to the mysterious concoction of chopped veal or some other undetermined species. He drew a huge laugh by saying, "As Harry Truman once said, 'If you can't stand the heat in the kitchen don't eat the meatloaf at the Shoreham Hotel.'" However, the Shoreham's meatloaf is Châteaubriand compared to the gravy-laden hockey pucks proudly served at some of the banquets of America. Rarely does one find any imagination used at all.

One exception that comes to mind was a stupendous affair at which I was the speaker. This is not to say that I made it imaginative, but what did make it different was that I felt I was dining with the Luftwaffe. The entire hall had been transformed into a German festival so authentic that it made you wonder who won the war. This was not some feeble American imitation Oktoberfest—no, this was a 12-course Bavarian board bender that would make Goering's mouth water: red cabbage and dumplings, schnitzel à la Holstein, potato soup, enough beer to float the *Bismarck*, all topped off with peppermint schnapps. It was accompanied by Mozart's more lively pieces rendered by tuba, trumpet, and trombone players in leather pants. The walls were festooned with eagles, flags, and iron crosses, and the entire effect made half the crowd want to invade Poland.

Let me add that this German orgy did not take place in Heidelberg, Munich, or even Pennsylvania. It was held in Savannah, Georgia. They hold it every year, and I doubt if there are enough people of German descent in that town to fill a VW station wagon, but who cares? It is something different. The only mistake at that entire affair was me. I bombed—upstaged by the food.

6) THE MUSIC. The proper selection of background music for a dinner falls somewhere between a single strolling violinist and the Marine Band trumpeting Sousa with a wind velocity that can blow the dishes off the table. A continental flavor is often sought in the choice of music, and the resulting continent can be Antarctica. The low-budget cheapies who set up a cash bar are usually the same ones who employ thrift in music.

One strolling violinist weaving in and out of the tables at a dinner for 2,000 is not only cheap, but hazardous duty for the violinist, when you consider that at least 1,500 of the guests want to hear

"Somewhere My Love" and the rest crave "Hot Canary" and can be downright hostile if they don't hear it. (You probably thought that the world was divided into two classes of people—those who dislike "Hot Canary" and those who detest it—but there is a "Hot Canary" Secret Society, and many a fiddler ignorant of that painful little piece has been found with his bow through his heart.)

The rhapsodizing violinist likewise poses a certain danger to the guests as he hovers over the table diligently drawing his bow across the strings. Flecks of rosin falling from the horsehair into the gravy can be unsettling. On second thought, at most banquets this accident can be an improvement, since the rosin can enhance the taste of the food far better than the genuine artificial flavoring already in the dish.

In Washington, military music is often played, particularly at the opening of a banquet. A color guard of four men, each representing a different branch of service, carries the flag up to the Head Table. They bring their rifles and bayonets to "present arms," and the National Anthem is played. This sort of pomp makes a nice impression on the out-of-towners, not only showing them where their defense dollars are going, but also because bayonets seem to whet the appetite.

It's amazing how many sexagenarians want to re-up after one of those color guard presentations. I've seen them leave their salads half-eaten as they rush from the table to the sound of snare drums. When the others inquire if old Harry went to the men's room, his deserted wife just says, "No, he went to join his old outfit at Saint Lo."

The playing of the National Anthem brings up another danger point in the progession of the banquet. As soon as the first notes are heard, what should be a surging feeling of patriotism often turns into a guilty awareness that very few are singing along. And those who are attempting to tackle this difficult song are doing a mighty poor job of it.

For quite some time now, there has been a growing movement to throw out the anthem and replace it with, perhaps, "America the Beautiful." This would be an improvement, but I doubt that many people would stand for it. If we ever did replace the "Star-Spangled Banner," I suppose it would be missed by the half-dozen opera singers who are able to get through it. The distance from the lowest to the highest note can only be traveled by anyone proficient in both "Asleep in the Deep" and "Indian Love Call."

An easier-to-sing anthem would be nice. We would all sing out, other nations would see how patriotic we are, and most important, banquets and ball games would get off to a more rousing start. So, what song should we use? I vote for "Send in the Clowns."

7) SPEECHES AND ENTERTAINMENT. Directly behind every Head Table, not seen by the audience, is another table holding a number of wooden or brass objects. They are trophies or plaques, or both. Count them and you'll know how many speeches there will be.

The purpose of the speeches is twofold: as acceptance of the award and as an endurance test for the audience. There the audience sits, filled to capacity with whiskey, white rolls, and chocolate mousse, at the mercy of the speakers who fill the air with electric utterances:

"Thank you, George, and thank you ladies and gentlemen for this undeserved award.

"What this plaque really says is that all of us in the National Association of Lawn Furniture Dealers have taken the bull by the horns, turned our backs to Big Brother, and let the chips fall.

"And it can't be done overnight. No, sir, it takes Bob in accounting, Ernie in marketing, and Betty—hey, let's not forget Betty (applause, applause), best little typist ever to come across the pike—the entire NALFD family—we're a team—and just like ol' Winston Churchill said, we'll fight them in the cities, we'll fight them in the streets and never surrender. And what else did Winnie say? I give you blood, sweat, and wicker chairs! Heh, heh."

Anyone engaged in one of the oldest professions in the world—public speaking for money—learns early in the game to beware of plaques. Exposure to plaques can be hazardous to one's health, because when a public speaker is given an award (which is a nicer word than "plaque"), it usually means that he isn't going to be paid, but rather that he is the one to be framed. All he gets is a piece of wood.

You can't eat a plaque. You might get a dollar for a plaque at a pawn shop. Nor is a plaque very decorative. About the only thing a plaque goes with is other plaques. So the next time you walk into a person's office, count the number of plaques on the wall and you'll know the number of times he has made a speech for free. Now if you have done something to deserve an award, or even won the Nobel Prize, you would be a cad to go and accept without making a speech of thanks. If you have discovered a cure for prickly heat or taught a goat to sing "You'll Never Walk Alone," you deserve recognition—go and accept the award, besides there might be money with it. (However, money is usually connected with the word "prize." Awards and plaques never are. Nobody ever heard of the Nobel Plaque. The moral is, if you owe somebody money, don't pay him—send him a plaque.)

The president of the United States is invited to just about every banquet held in Washington, but attends only a few, at which time he attempts humor in his speech. Jimmy Carter, who was not expected to join the Washington social whirl, surprised us when he not only attended some of the ritualistic dinners of the press, but scored some big laughs while doing so.

At the annual bash held by the White House correspondents, the head of the group, in his speech, chided Carter about the lack of women and blacks in his new administration. When it was Carter's turn to speak, he topped the newsman by saying that his administration was patterned after the Head Table at this particular dinner. At that moment, the thousand in attendance observed that the correspondents' Head Table included no women and that the only black had arrived with the president, since he was a Secret Service man! Sustained laughter.

A few months later Carter addressed the Urban League. The opening session of its convention was filled with charges that the new president was not doing enough for blacks. In attendance were the most celebrated blacks in the country, and at the time Alex Haley's book *Roots* was enjoying unprecedented success. The night of Carter's address, the president managed to increase the atmosphere of agitation by arriving an hour late. However, with a masterful touch, he improved the situation with his opening line: "I'm sorry I'm late tonight. About an hour ago I ran into Alex Haley in the lobby and I made the mistake of asking him how his family was."

Just before the Camp David peace talks in the fall of 1978, Jimmy Carter's standing in the polls was beginning to resemble the average temperature in Nome. Immediately after the talks, his popularity increased impressively, and he indicated as much in a speech he delivered in New Jersey. Looking out over the cheering, waving crowd, he said, "Well, it certainly is nice once again to see people holding up all five fingers."

The silent expletive of the protruding middle finger was also faced during the campaign of 1976 by Vice President Nelson Rockefeller. A group of young people standing right up front gave Rocky this obscene gesture. Rockefeller decided to fight fire with fire and gave the finger right back to them. An alert photographer preserved the moment for the ages. This, shall we say, informal picture of the vice president of the United States ranks with the raising of the flag on Iwo Jima in the annals of photojournalism. Actually, I always thought Rocky was merely demonstrating how his brother David turns down a loan at Chase Manhattan.

The safest kind of humor at any occasion is directed at oneself. Politicians, unless they are attacking their opponents in an election, chide themselves so that the folks will see what good sports they are.

Sometimes an attack on an opponent can be pretty funny without the intent. The Republicans in New York State brought me to Syracuse to cheer them up during the 1978 governor's race. Which they lost. Perry Duryea, the GOP candidate trying to oust Governor Hugh Carey, lashed out at Carey's record, building a crescendo leading up to the ultimate charge that "Hugh Carey is paid with taxpayer's money!" The fact that this is the way it's supposed to be was lost on the angry partisans who cried out, "No, this is an outrage!" I sat there chuckling within, wondering why, with such hilarity available, I was needed.

The finest example of the self-deprecating joke concerns the one told at a banquet by the popular Washington radio and TV personality Ed Walker. At this particular affair, I was being roasted at the National Press Club, and the speakers included UPI reporter Helen Thomas and Congressman Mo Udall, both of whom can turn a dreary banquet into a spritely affair.

Turning to me, Udall declared, "We're going to give this bastard a fair trial and then we're gonna hang him. We will abide by Jack Anderson's law which says, 'If you can't say something good about a fellow, then by God let's hear it.' "

Helen Thomas was a bit more kind as she reminded the audience that I had something in common with two presidents: "He plays the piano like Truman and the yo-yo like Nixon."

Included in the firing squad that evening was William Simon, who later became Nixon's Secretary of the Treasury. At the time, Simon was the so-called energy czar, and since the oil embargo and gas shortages were going on, he was catching a considerable amount of flak. For him even to show up at the National Press Club at such a time clearly demonstrated that Simon was one of the tough who gets going when the going gets tough. So to speak.

Deftly redirecting the fire aimed at him and pointing it toward me, Simon let go with this: "The real crisis in America today is a humor crisis. And Mark Russell is the man to blame. He and his cohorts are in a conspiracy, and they are going to force the public to pay more and more to keep hearing the same crude jokes. This absolutely represents a threat to our national levity. Russell is responsible for inflation. Just spend a few dollars to hear his act and you'll see how little money buys." Amusing. Faintly.

By the time it was Ed Walker's turn to speak, it seemed that he was in a pretty tough spot. Since Ed is blind, his speeches are written in Braille. After his few opening sentences, pretending to muff a line, he said, "Excuse me, folks, but just before the dinner a waiter stepped on my notes."

After Richard Nixon won the Vietnam war and brought our boys back home to peace with honor, the climate in Washington became a bit more relaxed. At an informal dinner, an off-the-record debate was scheduled between two men who had been bitter adversaries during the war years, Senator Frank Church and Secretary of State Henry Kissinger. Now that peace was at hand, just as Kissinger had promised, the debate was to be all in fun. Richard Nixon, for years, had been friends with several veteran comedy writers in Hollywood, and they were commissioned to help Kissinger write his speech. Senator Church, having lesser resources from which to draw, contacted me.

Now the problem with writing for these guys is that I can only imagine what jokes I would do in their particular circumstances; to put my words and attitudes into their mouths usually doesn't work. So I called an old friend from Washington, Jim Mulligan, who began his writing career on the landmark NBC show in the sixties, "Laugh In." As I described the Kissinger–Church debate to him, Jim stopped laughing long enough to tell me that he was one of the writers working on the Kissinger speech. So Mulligan and I, acting as double agents, manipulated the Kissinger–Church debate, tilting it toward Church. We had Senator Church saying things like, "I had a feeling you were going to say that, Henry, so let me just say . . ." Of course Church had no such feeling at all. I merely had him respond to Kissinger's material fed to me by one of his writers. I suppose that after that kind of experience, Mulligan and I could easily get a job writing snappy one-liners for both Sadat and Begin.

The roast, originally the ribald stag tradition of theatrical clubs such as the Lambs and the Friars, has been laundered for television and is now familiar to every household. I knew the idea of these insult-ridden spectacles had just about run its course when I received a call from a sweet-sounding lady who asked, "Mr. Russell, we need your help. We're having a little box supper here at Saint Anselm's and we wish to roast our pastor." I wondered if the good folks at St. Anselm's knew what an authentic roast was. Of course, if the pastor were to be given the kind of four-letter-sprinkled lambasting that was done prior to television, the congregation would face instant mass excommunication.

If you haven't yet grown weary of roasts and wish to rotate your pastor or anyone else on a skewer, I offer the following all-purpose roast recipe. All you need do is fill in the blanks; this formula should fit any victim:

> Good evening, ladies and gentlemen: We the (*name of organization*) are gathered together for the dubious task of honoring (*name of roastee*) even though he's our 1. (*boss*) 2. (*pastor*) 3. (*senator*) 4. (*leader in the community*). It is his inspiration that motivates us to do more than our best under fear of 1. (*unemployment*) 2. (*eternal damnation*) 3. (*being linked with him*) 4. (*public whipping*). I learned about the early life of (*roastee*) from the good people of (*roastee's birthplace*) where he was born on (*roastee's birthdate*), a (*roastee's astrological sign,*) who's Mercury was in the seventh house of Uranus. Those of you familiar with

astrology know that this is the same sign as Genghis Kahn and Ma Barker. I visited (*roastee's birthplace*) last weekend and was taken to his boyhood place of worship, the Shrine of Saint Attila. As a boy, little (*roastee*) dreamed of being a lovable (*roastee's occupation*). Well, one out of two isn't bad. (*Roastee*) came from a humble beginning which can only be matched by his humble ending. A reporter once asked him, "Mr. (*roastee's last name*), what is your reaction to this reputation you seem to have of being a 1. (*gut fighter*) 2. (*foot kisser*) 3. (*back stabber*) 4. (*horse thief*) 5. (*wife swapper*) 6. (*ogre*) 7. (*two-faced person*)?" (*Roastee's first name*) just looked at the reporter and 1. (*kicked him in the gut*) 2. (*kissed his foot*) 3. (*stabbed him in the back*) 4. (*stole his horse*) 5. (*swapped his wife*) 6. (*ogred*) 7. (*smiled and frowned*).

But let us turn back the pages of history. We find (*roastee*) as a fun-loving student in the little red school house in (*roastee's birthplace*), from which he was once expelled from biology class for using a karate chop on a defenseless toad. His quest for knowledge took him to that world-renowned institution of higher learning, the Warren G. Harding Municipal College of Piqua, Ohio, where he received his diploma for staying awake. After college he won a seat in the state legislature, where he soon championed the (*roastee*) Wilderness Act, named after the act he once committed in the wilderness. He often addressed himself to national issues, such as advocating a strong defense. And with his record he needed one. Actually the main reason he wanted to get into politics was because it was all indoor work with no heavy lifting. Which, incidentally, is the description of (*roastee's girlfriend's name*)'s first job.

But the truth is that (*roastee*) is not ruthless and not tough. No, he's gentle, he's a pussycat, he's a darling. Come to think of it, he's really a little effeminate. But no matter—his place in history is secure. For in time, all Americans will hear the echo of his words: "Remem-

ber me? This is (*roastee*) for American Express credit
cards."

During twenty years of attending banquets, I have had a recurring
dream. First, in my subconscious, I visualized the kind of banquet
I would design, but now I think about it when I'm awake. When I
sit half dozing at a Head Table listening to the speeches I think of
a better banquet world—a world where the banquet banalities
have been crushed, where the people are free, free at last from the
mundane unoriginal status quo of the organizational dinner. Yes, I
have a dream. Let me describe my imaginary banquet to end all
banquets.

To begin with, the reception is held in the boiler room of the
hotel. The subterranean levels of especially the older hotels are fascinating places. With a reception in the bowels of the building
there would be no painful attempts at making light cocktail chat-
ter. Everything down there is a conversation piece: "Say, that's an
interesting pile of mattresses over there—I wonder who's slept on
them." As the strolling trio—a bassoon, an oboe, and a glocken-
spiel—play selections from *Hair*, the guests, warmed by the
cheery furnace, unwind as they peruse the broken lamps, the
heaps of cracked shower curtains, and the vintage 1937 furniture.

Now, up to the ballroom for dinner. While the liver entreé is
still in the ovens the guests take their seats, all of which are at the
Head Table. The Head Table can easily accommodate everyone,
since it is the only table and it runs along the perimeter of the
room, lining the walls. The entire center is open, to be used for the
entertainment later. Everyone is arranged around the table, not
according to rank, position, or marital status, but according to
height. So that when the huge circle is closed, the tallest person is
sitting next to the shortest. Different.

Time for the invocation. During my long attendance at banquets I have spent a great deal of time with head bowed during
thousands of blessings before the meal. If you added up all that
time at prayer, I suppose I could rival the devotions of a Trappist
monk. I confess that during the more lengthy invocations, my
mind has drifted, wondering whether the clergyman will be honest
enough to say: "Heavenly Father, we thank Thee for the food,
which is getting cold because I'm droning on too long."

I have an interesting method of measuring the length of invocations. To look at your watch is not only suspicious, it also makes
you appear to be a wretched heathen. What I do is watch the salad
dressing. Thousand Island over hearts of lettuce is *de rigeur* at
these things, and I always compare the thick dressing's slow
progression sliding down the side of the heart of lettuce to the
length of the invocation. If the salad dressing wins, the clergyman
has been on too damn long.

If you are attending a banquet where the man of the cloth is a
Unitarian, you could be in luck. I have found the invocations of
Unitarians to be remarkably short. I suppose it's because at least
some of them aren't too sure to whom they are addressing their
prayer. A Unitarian clergyman, not wishing to offend, is liable to
stand at the Head Table, throw his arms heavenward, and cry out,
"To whom it may concern!" Whereupon everyone sits down and
digs in.

Now here is my plan for the all-purpose dream banquet-to-end-
all-banquets. For the invocation, you tell the clergyman privately
to keep praying until someone tells him to stop. If you can't find
one willing to go along with the gag, find a person unknown to the
crowd, hire an actor, or get someone to keep talking and see how
much time elapses before anybody musters up enough courage to
interrupt this ecclesiastical filibuster. How long would it be before
people started to giggle? A half hour? An hour? Who would take it
upon himself to tell a minister to knock it off? Days could go by.
Weeks. It would be a fascinating study of human behavior. Someday I'll do it.

As I mentioned, the main course at my banquet would be liver. I
happen to adore liver and the serving of it to several hundred people would be the most significant event in the history of dining
since Marie Antoinette said, "Let them eat Sara Lee."

Another tradition that would bite the dust at my event would be
the dessert parade. Hotels take pride in arming the waiters with
sparklers stuck into the baked Alaska as they parade into the darkened room. It has the effect of the Romans storming the temple in
an old Cecil B. DeMille movie.

I'd keep the parade, but not for the dessert. It would be a procession for the side dish. Sparklers would be stuck into the vegetable
in the Grand Okra Parade. As the band (fifty accordians and fifty

trumpets) played the Sabre Dance, the waiters carrying the okra, with swords strapped to their sides, would storm the Head Table, unsheath their weapons, and, pointing them menacingly at the guests' throats, would sneer, "You haven't touched your liver!"

At last the dinner is over, and it's time for the show. I have thought long and hard about the perfect choice of entertainment. The show area is in the center of the ballroom surrounded by the table. In this space I would place three large circus rings.

In the first ring, to kick off the show, I'd put George C. Scott in full cavalry uniform to deliver his stirring opening speech from *Patton.* He is soon joined by Anita Bryant and they sing "Battle Hymn of the Republic" in perfect two-part harmony. She is surrounded by a dozen chorus boys prancing in nothing but feathers and a G-string.

In the next ring we have a dramatic contrast—100 guys in chains singing "Let My People Go" as Charles Colson is lowered from the ceiling, illuminated by a pin spotlight, and blesses them, with one hand placed on his best-selling book. As a backdrop, a screen descends on which there is a huge blow-up of the Watergate apartments.

The third ring is where we find the real action—the verbal gladiators. In a frenzied spectacle, Jeane Dixon, Jimmy the Greek, Louis Harris, Elmo Roper, and George Gallup shout fearful predictions at each other at a rapid pace. Louder and louder, faster and faster, the doomsaying accelerates. One prophecy after the other, statistics, opinions, surmises, conjectures, all machine-gunned at the fighters until only one remains standing and becomes the victor, the others having succumbed to deep depression and silence.

The action in the three rings is simultaneous and leaves the audience totally sated. And so my dream banquet is over—a total and ultimate experience removing the desire of anyone in the audience to attend another. For this one cannot be topped.

But I know in my heart that such an event will never be, and perhaps it is just as well, because if all banquets were to come to an end, perhaps that would signify the end of a great status symbol of the American middle class. And, not incidentally, the disappearance of a major source of my income.

So let them live—Viva Banquets! Long live the Head Table, glory to the salads, good tidings to the string beans. Come let us praise the chicken. All hail to outgoing presidents, as we bow our heads for the benediction: "We thank thee for this, the closing banquet of our convention. Watch over us until next year when we meet in Seattle. We ask for a reasonable margin of profit, and deliver us from excess regulation. Amen."

I guess I've been pretty rough on this great American tradition. Perhaps so, but secretly I love to attend them. Besides, my food bill is next to nothing.